# CONTROL YOUR EATING

*A Behaviourist Speaks*

**A Step Towards Successful Dieting and Fighting Obesity**

**Richard M. Sanders, PhD**
**Consulting Psychologist**

Railroad Street Press
St. Johnsbury, VT

Printed in the United States of America


Cover Design by Susanna Walden


LIBRARY OF CONGRESS
CATALOGING-IN-PUBLICATION DATA
_____

Sanders, Richard M., PhD.


ISBN  978-1-936711-20-8

Railroad Street Press
394 Railroad St., Ste 2
St. Johnsbury, VT 05819
railroadstreetpress.com

Dedicated to

**ALL THOSE WHO WISH TO TAKE CONTROL**

to my mentors

Edward J. Green then at Dartmouth College

Marcus B. Waller then at UNC Chapel Hill

and to their mentor

B F Skinner

**Table of Contents**

# Control Your Eating: The Behaviourist Speaks

## *A Step Towards Successful Dieting and Fighting Obesity*

### Introduction

In this manual, I offer the reader (that's you) a number of "tricks" for changing your eating behaviour. These tricks are based upon sound principles of behaviour. These tricks are easy to understand and very easy to use. Of course, "breaking the rules" which these tricks imply, is equally easy to do.

So, it is really in the end all up to you to decide if you are going to **be honest with yourself**. I cannot help you with that potential problem. I can however offer you many "hints" and "tricks" which, if you are serious about taking yourself in hand and controlling your eating behaviour, will help you greatly.

I call these ideas **"tricks"** because I strongly suspect that most of you will say, of most of these ideas, that "they are obvious" and "anyone could think them up". You are of course absolutely right. These tricks are no more than common sense and the moment you read each, you will wonder why you did not think of doing that before.

### About Behavioural Psychology

There are no deep secrets about behavioural psychology. The basics remain terribly simple and extremely powerful. There are really very few "rules" of behaviour. Here are the most important.

**Rule Number One:** If you do something and have a pleasant outcome, then you are more likely to do that again (positive feedback).

**Rule Number Two:** If you do something which results in an unpleasant outcome, you are less likely to do that again (negative feedback).

**Rule Number Three:** The sooner the "outcome" happens after you do what you do, the more likely that you will or will not do that again (time of feedback).

## About Eating Behaviour.

Eating is a behaviour just like any other behaviour and subject to these same rules. However, eating is most subject to Rule Number One with the feedback being almost immediate. That is, when we eat, we are immediately pleased by taste. If we pay attention to our food, we may also be immediately pleased with the sight of the food, the aroma coming from the food, and the textures in our mouth.

All of these factors are the enemy of those who eat too much, too often, and too fast. And it is usually the case that these three behavioural factors are what contribute hugely to our being overweight.

**Eating too much** means we take in too many calories and thus give our body an excess over what it needs to maintain a healthy weight.

**Eating too often** usually means we are snacking throughout the day and this just increases our overeating as well as strengthens our overeating habit.

**Eating too fast** means that even when our body might signal us that it has had enough, we jam a lot in before the body really has time to force that signal through to our attention.

Of course there is another factor which makes us overweight and this is also a matter of our behaviour. And it falls under the same rules as any other behaviour. **This factor is our choice of foods**. Why do we like what we like? See Rule Number One!!! Most often it is taste and taste most frequently relates to the very food items which we are least likely to be able to take in without having weight problems: **fats, sugar, and salt. (the big three of our eating problems).** Why do we like fries, pulled pork, hamburgers, deep fried corn dogs, and broasted whatevers? As a noted chef once said to me, "fat is the chef's friend". Why do we like chocolate, gum drops, cookies of all kinds, and most every dessert we can imagine? Why do we like peanuts, potato chips, and those "snack bars"? See Rule Number One and Rule Number Three: they taste great!!! They provide an immediate and pleasant experience. So the more we eat from the big three, the more we "like" them and the greater becomes our problem of eating and weight control.

## In summary

It is obvious that Rules Number One and Three rule the world of our eating. It is also obvious that Rule Number Two fails to change our behaviour because of Rule Number Three: the unpleasant result of our behaviour is not immediately obvious. In fact, it is so remote from our eating that we often truly fail to see the relationship between eating and weight gain in any sense but the truly intellectual one. We "know" what we are doing to ourselves as we stuff in yet another of the "big three", but we do not have the reality of the effect like we do the immediate positive feedback. Thus **Rules Number One and Three, cooperating with "the big three", win again!**

Thus it is a matter of learning to impose self control over your eating behaviour and it is this area in which you (yes, back to you) need help. It is for that purpose that this manual is written for you. The "tricks" are designed to help you learn ways to block some of your old habits in order for Rule Number One to help you. I have provided you with ways to feel good about what you are doing. It may not taste, smell, or feel as good as the results of eating do, but it is better than nothing and depends upon you, as a thinking person, to **be able to say to yourself, "that's good" or "you are doing the right thing", or "OK"!** These statements by themselves can help, and as the immediate results of your behaviour (Rule Number Three), they can be very supportive of your new behaviour.

Two kinds of "tricks" are offered: those which block your inappropriate eating behaviour and those which provide you a way to keep track of your eating behavior. Keeping track generally means just making a mark on a chart. It is making this mark which allows you to feel good about what you are doing. Charting your behaviour also gives you the opportunity to look at your past behaviour and again feel good about what you are doing for yourself. Seeing yourself comply with "blocking tricks" and charting your progress allow you to **feel good immediately by telling yourself how "good" you are being and becoming.**

So here you go!! The sections of this manual take you through many aspects of your eating problems and provide you with methods for dealing with each. Beyond providing "blocks" and "charts", my role as your behavioural leader is done. It is up to you to make use of these materials to your advantage. It is solely on you to do the work that all of this represents. **No one can force you but you!!** If you try what is offered, you will be doing it for you. Others may help you by invoking Rule Number One when you show them what you are doing: especially if your weight chart shows success. But **remember, it is you who is working for you.**

Good luck and best wishes from your behaviourist.

# HOW TO USE THIS MANUAL

## If you did not read the Introduction, this is a must!!

I suggest that the best way for you to start using this manual is to look over the index of topics. There are many topics and some may only be useful to you at special times. But you probably should start by scanning this list so that you will know what is available to you.

Your second step might best be taken by reading some of the sections which seem of the greatest interest or relevance to you. Some make fairly obvious starting places, such as <u>Weight Charting,</u> <u>Goal Setting for Caloric Intake</u>, <u>Goal Setting for Weight Loss</u>, and <u>Food Values</u>. Some may have special interest for you, such as <u>Promises, Resolutions, and Other Potential Lies</u>, <u>Moods</u>, and <u>Proper Nutrition: USDA Style</u>.

> **NOTE**: Every time a section of this manual is cited or referred to, it is underlined. That may help you remember to use or seek out materials which you have not yet used.

Wherever you start, you will quite naturally move from there through much of the rest of the manual as you define your own needs and recognize your own habits (bad behaviour). Thus, over time, you will probably wish to read most of the sections. Of course, you may read all of the sections at the outset in order to have a full picture of what is available and where you and your needs fit in. You may even discover some things about yourself which you did not know until they became obvious in the section.

The Appendix to this manual contains the charts which you may wish to use. Do not get overwhelmed by all these charts. You will most likely want to slowly break yourself into the routine of charting. Probably the weight chart is the best place to start and then gradually expand your record keeping as you become used to the process. The process of charting is designed to give you the opportunity to experience that positive feedback (Rule Number One).

So it is up to you. I have ordered the sections to reflect some general sense of an order which might serve some of you: especially for the first three sections. Beyond those, please do not feel that the order I have selected is necessarily meant as somehow the "most sensible" or "most logical" order.

And finally, **please enjoy!**

# A Note About Dieting and Diets

Most of you who have purchased this manual will be interested in dieting to lose weight (Some perhaps to gain and some to maintain). Since most of you are probably interested in weight loss, the remainder of my comments are directed to that end. To me there are no secrets about dieting. Regardless of the "name" of your diet it is a very straightforward matter.

**The formula for weight loss is simple.**

## Calories taken in must be less than calories used up!

Exercise spends calories. I have yet to read or hear of a comparative study of diets which does not in the end say that the only systematic weight loss factor was **exercise**.

With regard to the diets themselves apart from exercise, I am a firm believer in a balanced diet. Emphasizing one kind of intake to the exclusion or near exclusion of another makes absolutely no sense to me. Of course, being the husband of a nutritionist, I may have picked up a bias somewhere along my fifty years of this exposure. My wife has contributed the basics for some of the sections of this manual. She also points out why some of these special diets are in fact potentially dangerous to your health. (See <u>Proper Nutrition: USDA Style</u>.)

There are many books on dieting. Most all acknowledge that dieting is difficult. People tend to lose and then gain the weight back--- and sometimes more. Most authors acknowledge that dieters reach plateaus from which further weight loss seems impossible. These authors generally agree that plateaus reflect the fact that the body is adjusting and that you need to "wait it out". (See <u>Goal Setting for Weight Loss</u>.)

The important factor in this manual is that you are learning to **<u>control your eating behaviour</u>**. Once you are in control of your behaviour, you need not worry about regaining the weight you have lost. Diets only help you as long as you stay on them. **Changing your behaviour leaves you with habits which last beyond a diet.** Thus this manual focuses on **<u>learning to eat appropriately</u>** rather than on dieting <u>per se</u>.

# Weight Charting

If you are like many people, you have a great capacity for fooling yourself. Even when we have direct evidence of what we are doing, we often choose to ignore it, disbelieve it, or fail to attend to it—especially if it does not agree with what we want to hear, see, or otherwise acknowledge. I think this is especially true for those who are dieting to lose weight. If we cut back on even a single meal, we feel we have contributed significantly to our weight loss. And we remember that meal and use it as the basis for rationalizing a half dozen other meals or snacks which put us over our diet intake limit.

So here is the **TRICK**. Chart your weight. The act of charting gives you the chance to feel good if your weight has decreased and to ask yourself "why" if it has not. Daily charting is better than weekly because weekly charting violates the best of Rule Number Three. And you will not be disappointed or discouraged by discovering that you did not lose weight after a week of what you "thought" was a "good try".

This charting is simple. The chart I have provided you is easy to read and score. The days are along the bottom of the chart. Along the side you must put a range of weights that includes your current weight at the top and your goal weight (see Goal Setting for Weight Loss) at the bottom with regular intervals in between. Choose the intervals between these two points so that it is easy to see that you have lost a single pound. That is, make the intervals which represent a single pound no smaller than two of the marks on the side of the chart. If the chart then is not big enough to represent your current weight and eventual goal weight, set an intermediate goal weight for the period of time for which the chart is designed. A sample chart is shown below.

## Sample Weight Chart

| Weight | | | | | | | | | | | | | | | | | | | | | | | | | | | | | | | |
|---|---|---|---|---|---|---|---|---|---|---|---|---|---|---|---|---|---|---|---|---|---|---|---|---|---|---|---|---|---|---|---|
| 195.5 | * | * | | | | | | | | | | | | | | | | | | | | | | | | | | | | | |
| 195.0 | | | * | * | * | | | | | | | | | | | | | | | | | | | | | | | | | | |
| 194.5 | | | | | | * | | | | | | | | | | | | | | | | | | | | | | | | | |
| 194.0 | | | | | | | * | * | * | | | | | | | | | | | | | | | | | | | | | | |
| 193.5 | | | | | | | | | | * | * | * | | | | | | | | | | | | | | | | | | | |
| etc | | | | | | | | | | | | | * | * | | | | | | | | | | | | | | | | | |
| | M | T | W | T | F | S | S | M | T | W | T | F | S | S | | | | | | | | | | | | | | | | |

Days

Each day, you must plot your weight on this chart by putting a dot over the day at the level of your weight. You will have to use a number of these charts over time so extra copies have been provided in the Appendix.

The most difficult part of this will be getting your weight. Unless you are going to buy a fine set of electronic scales, you will find that all scales are not born equal. Even from moment to moment they may not give the same result. Here are some tips which will help make your measurements more accurate.

- Try to stand in the same place on the scales each time you weigh yourself. Leaning forward or back may change the outcome so test this and then choose how you will stand from then on.
- Try to keep the scales in exactly the same place for each weighing.
- Try to weigh yourself at the same time in your daily schedule—before or after Breakfast for example. Remember, a glass of juice or water weighs nearly a half of a pound.
- Try to schedule your bowel movement time to be either before or after weighing so that it is the same each day.
- If you have to violate the points above, you may wish to skip the charting for that day—or chart and see the effect of the violation.

If you live very near a physician's office, and know the receptionist or nurse, perhaps you might be allowed to get your daily weighing there. The physician's scales are generally very accurate.

Let charting become a habit. Each time you chart your weight you may get a good feeling from the weight loss you see and you can also remind yourself that you are doing a good thing for yourself—**gaining a good habit—not more weight!!**

# Goal Setting for Caloric Intake

How many calories a day are right for you? This is a really big and can be a somewhat complex issue. But there are some simple ways to look at it.

1. How many calories are you taking in now?

2. How many calories are you using now?

The answer to these two questions can tell you where to set your daily caloric intake limit. Here are the steps to answer the two questions.

1. Do a food recall for about three days. Record all the foods you have eaten including how much of each. This is easier than you think. That candy bar has its nutritional characteristics right on the wrapper. The cereal box does too. So do the wrappers on most prepackaged food products. (See Food Values) Total all the calories you took in during each of the each three days. Add the three days together and divide by three. This is the average number of calories you take in per day. This is the answer to the first question.

2. There are numerous charts out to tell you the caloric value of almost all daily activities. (See Activity Charting.) From sex to standing around looking off into the distance, these values can be determined and you can count up a fairly accurate picture of your daily output. Do this for three days; add all the calories worn off for each day. Add the three days value together and divide by three. This will give you the average daily calories worked off. This is the answer to the second question.

Now your decisions are very direct ones. But I cannot dictate the outcome to you. You have three basic choices.

1. You can decrease your caloric intake to match your caloric output.

2. You can increase your caloric output to match your caloric intake by doing more active things.

11

3. You can do both at once. Set the caloric level to one which might satisfy your need for food and increase your activity level so that you are using up that same level of calories.

I suspect that most of you will select the third alternative and it is probably the most sensible. As you become used to the idea of controlling your eating and becoming aware of your activity level (see Activity Charting) you may wish to change one or the other or both. For example, you may wish to increase your activity level so that you may take in more to eat (and still maintain or lose weight).

So set your caloric intake goal, determine how much activity you will engage in, and start your Weight Chart to see how you are doing. I expect that the feedback you get will be very positive.

# Goal Setting for Weight Loss

There are three primary methods of setting a goal for weight loss. They are equally good or bad depending upon how they affect you if you fail to meet the expectations.

The most simple is to set no goal at all and just see what happens when you control some aspects of your eating. Select a few modules from this manual and follow them while charting your weight over a few weeks. Then ask yourself if this is a sufficiently fast weight loss to make you happy about your progress—happy enough that is to continue. (Rule Number One.) You can then take on more controls from other modules if you wish or feel you need to.

Sometimes the primary motivation for losing weight is to fit into smaller size clothes. Another way to say that is that **"I want to look thinner"**. Hoping to throw away the "oversized" clothing in favor of smaller versions is a great motivator. The problem is that it may take so long to get to the goal that unless you establish intermediate goals, you may quite likely lose interest. (Rule Number Three) The weight chart is one way of keeping track often enough to remain motivation. (See <u>Weight Charting</u>.)

Probably the most common method of setting a goal is to set a specific amount to be lost over some period of time. This is then divided by the period of time to give you a weekly loss rate. The danger here is that you may set too high a rate of loss and become too discouraged to continue after but a few weeks. **DO NOT SET YOURSELF UP FOR FAILURE!!** Again, it is the weight charting which will help you. Charting is easy and weight is reliably and easily measured. Be sure to read the section on <u>Weight Charting</u>.

No matter what kind of goal structure you use, **the process of weight loss is something you must understand.** We do not tend to lose weight at the same rate from week to week. Generally, we can expect to lose more as soon as we take steps to control our eating and then the process slows down. This is usually due to the body using up extra water before starting to use up excess fat. The guidelines below should help you understand the process and this understanding should in turn help protect you from setting too high a standard of loss. Thus you will be protected from a failure of Rule Number One.

The process of weight loss is generally seen as having five stages. These stages are slightly different for men and women.

**For men:**

An initial loss of about 4-5% over a 5-10 day period.

A 5-15 day period of minor weight loss: 0.5-1% per week.

An 8-12 week period of moderate weight loss: 1-1.5% per week.

A 10-20 day period of minor weight loss: 0.5-1% per week.

A long stretch of moderate weight loss until the goal is reached: 1-2% per week.

**For Women:**

An initial loss of about 2-3% over a 5-10 day period.

A 5-15 day period of minor weight loss: 0.5% per week.

An 8-12 week period of moderate weight loss: 1-1.5% per week.

A 10-20 day period of minor weight loss: 0.5% per week.

A long stretch of moderate weight loss until the goal is reached: 1-1.5% per week.

Knowing that the process varies over time in this way, and following your weight chart, will make for both appropriate expectations and the positive feedback required to support your continuing to learn to **control your eating behaviour.**

# Food Values

There is an excellent source for determining the "value" of almost any food. This is the book by Bolles and Church entitled: <u>Food Values of Portions Commonly Used</u>, published by Lippincott Williams & Wilkins, eighteenth edition. The good news is that this is very complete. The bad news is that it is really quite expensive. But there is more good news: you can probably find it in most libraries.

The value of any food has many aspects. Most importantly for you, there are three major areas to which you will want to pay attention. Each food item has a certain number of calories associated with it for a specific amount of that food. When you think of some items which are low in calories, you must also realize that your choice of portion size will determine just how many calories you are taking in. "Pigging out" on a "low calorie" item such as only four chicken nuggets can result in a very high caloric intake. **Is that within your caloric intake goals?** (see <u>Goal Setting – Caloric Intake</u>.) Four such nuggets cost 210 calories. The 8 you are much more likely to eat either while snacking or for a meal will cost you 420 calories. That may be about one third of your daily allotment of calories. **Is that worth it?** Trying to starve later in that day in order to "make up" for this error is a risky business indeed.

The second area of great concern to you will be the nutritional value of the food. Some foods, such as popcorn, are virtually empty of nutritional value. Bolles and Church show that 1 cup with Pop Secret instead of butter has only 35 calories, 2.5 g fat, 1.0 g protein, 4.0 g carbohydrates, 60 mg of sodium and 10 mg potassium. But **beware** when you add regular butter and that large sprinkle of salt. The calorie count climbs rapidly and the salt will make you eat more.

Thirdly, some foods are absolutely loaded. It has been mentioned before that a very fine primary source for finding this information is Bolles and Church. This source gives the data for calories and nutrition on nearly every food you might run into. It is a little complicated to use so I will walk you through a food item using the tables found in the book.

Many of us love the taste of avocado, and especially when it is served as a dip for chips. Let's look at this food item. Of course the guacamole is bad enough: but adding the chips can make the calorie count even much worse. And what about the nutritional value of the chip? The avocado certainly has value but the chips add nothing but two of the big three enemies: fat and salt.

Florida Raw Avocado (From Bolles and Church)

| K Cal | H2O | Pro | CHO | SUGR | DFIB |
|-------|-------|-----|------|------|------|
| 340 | 242.4 | 4.8 | 27.1 | -0- | 16.1 |

| WT | FAT | SFA | MUFA | PUFA | CHOL |
|-----|------|-----|------|------|------|
| 304 | 27.0 | 5.3 | 14.8 | 4.5 | -0- |

## How about that for more than you ever wished to know!!!

In case you are still interested, here is the code.

*K CAL=calories. This is probably the most important for you.*
*H20=water          PRO=protein          CHO=carbohydrates*
*SUGR=sugar          DFIB=-dietary fiber          WT=weight*
*FAST=fat          SFA=saturated fatty acids*
*MUFA=monounsaturated fatty acids          SCHOL=cholesterol*

## Wow! Look at all that information.

When you think about the USDA 2005 food pyramid, there all the ingredients are listed for each of the food groups (see Proper Nutrition: USDA Style).

So where does an avocado fit into your diet? At 340 calories it is probably not a fit. But half of one does have only 170 calories and does have many other positive aspects such as DFIB, PRO, and CHO.

Now it is up to you. How deeply you want to get into the food value business depends really on how important all of this is to you. You can lose weight without paying much attention to the complexity of food values, but the more you do know, the better off you and your body may be. A proper diet such as that of the USDA 2005 pyramid is scientifically sound. Knowing that you are eating what is good for you as well as what is appropriate for your weight control should most certainly make you feel good about yourself (Rule Number One.)

# And finally, there is more good news!!

**If this is all just too much for you, then see the section on Snack Foods where you will find much of the same information is to be found on the labels of most if not all food packaging.**

# Beware The Fad Diets

Proper Nutrition: USDA Style

It is not the purpose of this manual to delve into the details or even concepts of the many fad diets that have come down the pike. Suffice it to say that almost all have the same two weaknesses.

First, they almost always result in weight loss closely followed by weight gain. For whatever reason, most people who try such a diet do so for only a moderate period of time—just long enough to make some modest weight loss before they tire of the diet's restrictions. They then gain back what they lost and sometimes even gain more. Stories of this outcome are frequent and even common within the same individual. One result is often that the person becomes so discouraged they just give up trying. This usually results in yet further weight gain and can lead to even greater medical and psychological problems such as diabetes, coronary disease, and depression, to name just a few.

Second, and probably of greater potential importance, is the fact that there is really no research literature to suggest that some of these fad diets are safe. Restricting your intake to just certain categories of food, starving yourself with appetizer suppressors, or taking in just one source of foods may not be a very healthy approach to the problem. In fact, some of these fads may be very hazardous to human health by not providing the distribution of foods which research seems to prove to be best for the human system.

It is strongly suggested here that you pay significant attention to the intake structure proposed by the United States Department of Agriculture. This so-called "pyramid" of food groups is an excellent source for helping you to understand what the human digestive, structural, nervous, and glandular systems need for proper functioning. Further, with care and planning on your part, you can achieve this properly balanced intake within almost any caloric level you impose upon yourself. (see Goal Setting – Caloric Intake.)

According to the USDA 2005 guidelines, our daily intake should include the following:

*3 servings of dairy products*
*9-13 servings of fruits and vegetables*
*3 servings of whole grains*

*(plus 2 servings of fish per week)*

But it is really more complicated than this. The actual number of servings really depends upon whether you are male or female and what your age and weight are. By going to the USDA Website <MyPyramid.gov – Inside the Pyramid>, you can enter these personal statistics and the system will display your actual suggested number of servings. Print this out and you have your guidelines against which to pose your personal food preferences.

There are many other websites you can find which offer ideas for menus, recipes, substitute ingredients, and other helpful information for you, the dieter. But I strongly feel that all should be taken in the context of this USDA "pyramid" and your overall weight control program.

# Snacking

## Beware the Munching Mouth

The idea of snacking is mentioned many times throughout the sections of the manual. It is an especially important issue for those of you trying to control your eating behaviour while at the same time preparing food for others. It is even more difficult if you are preparing" snack food" for others (see Snack Foods). Especially if your intake volume is low, the urge to snack to fill your stomach is very strong.

In general, snacking represents a great hazard to you because it is probably a "habit". You are probably used to snacking wherever and whenever. And most snacks are not foods you probably have on your eating schedule. They tend to be sweet and calorie/fat laden. Statistics show that the majority eat two snacks between meals and before going to bed.

Finally, let's face the facts. Snacking is eating.

## I must digress with a short story.

Many years ago I served as an assistant on a research project having to do with weight control. We took food recalls from our subjects and, with the help of a dietician, most were loosing weight gradually. Two were not however. In fact they continued to gain. I happened to be in a local eatery in mid afternoon and who was there having gummy goo rolls and coffee with heavy cream? You know who! The next time they came in for food recalls it was at once noted that this "snack" at mid day was not on their recall sheet at all. They were however, following all the rest of the prescriptions for their intake. When confronted, they both made us understand that this was "gnashing", a behaviour not counted as eating as it is loosely translated to mean "eating that does not matter (or count)". On further questioning, they both admitted to engaging in "gnashing" at least twice during each day and before going to bed (snack). Thus the mystery of their weigh gain was solved.

So what can you do? A few suggestions are offered and have been described as **TRICKS** in other sections.

1. Do not keep snacks around the house. (see The Kitchen.)
2. Do not purchase snacks. (see Shopping Techniques.)
3. Put leftovers out of sight, out of range, in difficult places to

easily get to (see <u>Leftovers</u>.)

4. No matter what your diet, there will be items which you are allowed to eat in large quantity (see <u>Food Values</u>.) Prepare a lot of this "appropriate snack" and make it easy to find. But be sure to eat it where it is appropriate to eat (see <u>Where to Eat</u>.)
5. Take your own snacks with you if necessary (see <u>Celebrations, Sprees, and Socials</u>.)

But again, let's face the facts. You may not be living alone.

You probably have to prepare food for others. They may eat more than you and have little interest in controlling their eating behaviour even if they support you in your effort (see <u>Support People and OTHERS</u>.) Giving them larger portions for regular meals is not that difficult. But providing for their "Munching Mouths" or need (wish for) snacks can be a problem.

If you have to prepare snacks for others in your house, then do so. But put them away were they are not a temptation for you and yet available to those in need.

**TRICKS.**

1. Label the snacks to identify the person for whom they are intended: kids and friends, etc. That way you are reminded that these snacks are not for you.
2. Ask others to eat their snacks somewhere out of your sight, sound, and smell range if possible. The last thing you need is to hear the crunch, smell the aroma, and see the snack disappearing into someone else's mouth.

### Some final notes

Snacking is a habit. Snacking is eating. Eating is what you are trying to control. So snacking throughout the day, even if you choose "appropriate snacks", is contributing to the habit. So try to minimize the snacking and make it a fixed time and place so that the habit does not spread itself all around the house and the clock.

You can use the <u>Master Chart</u> in the Appendix to note four things. First, the number of snack periods you had in a day. Second, if you ate appropriate snack materials. Third, if you ate them in the appropriate place. And forth, how many snack opportunities did you turn down. You can certainly make yourself feel good using this chart when you see improvement.

It is a reality that we live in a world of snacks and snacking. But limiting the opportunity to snack is very important. And yet there are times when a snack is an expected part of an activity. A TV party is an example. Card parties almost always require a snack if not an outright dessert. What to do?

Your choice of snack or dessert will be very important. (see <u>Snack Foods</u> and <u>Celebrations, Sprees, and Socials</u>.)

# Snack Foods

We live in a world of snack foods or fast food. We are awash in all kinds of food in our world but snack foods are in many ways the greatest of our enemies for losing weight. They are constantly available. They are packaged for convenience. And they almost always taste great for they almost always have all three of our biggest enemies: fat, sugar, and salt (see Introduction.)

The good news is that the government requires these items to be labeled with a list of ingredients. Usually the amount per serving of each ingredient is listed. Sometimes, ingredients are only listed in order from most to least. If salt is listed first, it is the most common ingredient.

## READ THE LABELS

If you choose to buy the prepackaged items, read the information. Make sure they fit into your overall eating requirements. And perhaps you should take a refresher course from the sections on Snacking or Proper Nutrition: USDA Style. Here are some guidelines for selecting prepackaged foods which you might consider. The labels are a little tricky because you must be certain you have taken note of what the "serving size" is. All the values (percentages and grams) are based on that serving size. And these servings seem especially small in most of these snack foods.

### Remember the old ad?
### "Bet you can't eat just one!"

There is a reason they could make that statement. These snacks are designed to taste so good that you cannot help yourself but to eat them—and probably far more than a "single serving".

### Two Examples of the Bad and Ugly

A corn tostadas package shows that the "serving size" is I tostadas. This thin, four and a half inch disc is **bad enough by itself at 60 calories—** just think what the three or four you will probably eat if you get started will cost you and your diet.

A cookie designed for the "healthy" food market brags of no hydrogenated oil, dairy, or eggs products. On reading the label we find this four plus oz cookie is **two servings of 240 calories each, 90 of which are fat. The ugly cookie indeed!!**

## The Alternatives

There are snack foods which are good for you. In fact, there are many. But not very many of them come in the prepackaged condition seen in the convenience or grocery stores. Here are some thoughts on foods you can prepare for yourself as snacks when you need them (see Celebrations, Sprees, and Socials.)

Almost every vegetable can be eaten raw and most are very healthy indeed.

All colors of peppers, celery, carrots, beets, cauliflower, turnip, parsnip, sweet potato, jicama, and even the dreaded broccoli are all very tasty and very nutritious but without large calorie content. To make these vegetables even more interesting, don't just put out a plate of one kind. Mix them up so that there is a variety of colors and tastes.

## And lose the dip!
(unless you check out the cost to your program and find it safe.)

Instead of the standard store dips, try making up a salsa of your own. The ingredients are themselves nutritious and the spicing and use of herbs makes this kind of dip a great flavor addition to your raw vegetable offerings. You can even make a cracker to go with this dip. Here is a recipe for you to try.

## Crispy seeded crackers.
Using a whisk, mix 3 cups of flour, 1-1/4 teaspoons of salt, ½ teaspoon of baking powder, 2/3 cup of toasted sesame seeds, and 1 teaspoon freshly ground black pepper. After mixing, stir in 2 tablespoons of olive oil and then add 1 cup of water mixing until the dough is uniform. Divide the dough to make as many of the size cracker you wish and let rest while covered for 15 minutes. Roll out very thin and bake on a greased or parchment lined baking sheet at 450 deg. for about 6 minutes, then turn them over and finish baking (about 4 minutes). They should be nicely browned when done. Let them cool and then store in airtight containers until used.

Most fruits can be eaten raw and many of these are not only very nutritious but are not overly filled with calories---and certainly not with fats (check out Food Values section.)

Apples, peaches, pears, grapes, cherries, strawberries, watermelon, oranges, and grapefruit are all excellent choices.

**Note that these are to be eaten**
# <u>Raw</u>

**not as the processed products found in cans and jars with those wonderfully sweet-tasting syrups.**

Most of all, give your munching mouth something good to eat but without the risk of increasing your caloric intake.

**HINT**: By keeping food items like these in the refrigerator so that when the urge hits they are already for you, **you put a strong road block up against finding some other kind of snack—your enemies!!**

# Leftovers

Leftovers are almost always a great problem in our eating behaviour. They are "available food". They are often the main target of "snacking" along with other available foods such as cookies and crackers from the see-through containers on the kitchen shelf or counter top. They are an open invitation to "snack".

Yet leftovers seem to be an inevitable outcome of preparing food. Often, too much is put on the plate so that there is no leftover. Other times the serving bowl or platter is taken to the table with the "leftovers" (family style) immediately available at the table. And finally, leftovers are left in the kitchen and are consumed when you clear the dishes and "put away the leftovers".

If leftovers are allowed to come about at all (see Shopping Techniques), then something must be done so that they do not enter your food chain. Here are some blocking **TRICKS** you can use.

1. Do not prepare more food than you have determined to be the appropriate amount for each person being served (see Portion Size.) Thus there will be no leftovers.
2. Serve the food onto the plates or into the bowls **in the kitchen**. Then take them to the table. Therefore there are no "extra" portions on the table.
3. Put all leftovers away before you serve the table. Then you will not return to the kitchen after the meal and be faced with the temptation of those leftovers.
4. Do not put serving dishes on the table.
5. Package the leftovers in storage containers and put them away. Then they are not so easily available. This gives you some time to think about what you are doing if you start to give in and open the cabinet or refrigerator door.
6. Throw out the leftovers. This is a drastic measure to be used only as a last resort. There may be a long range benefit to this "blocking trick". By throwing away this extra food you may be sufficiently offended by the waste that you will change you purchasing habits (see Shopping Techniques.)

Packaging leftovers for storage is the most common and preferred method. Store them so that they are hard to get to, so that they do not constantly give off their aromas, and so that they are not seen. Then add the idea of making them hard to get to by putting them into containers which require significant effort to open. Containers with a good seal or jars with tight lids will make a difference.

Here are some additional **TRICKS**.
1. Place in back of refrigerator or cabinet.
2. Use opaque containers.
3. Label as "leftover" and specify when they will next appear and /or for whom they are being stored.

***But if you cannot control your search for food such as leftovers,***

# *then throw them out.* *If you are so uncontrolled that you must dive into the garbage after them, please refer yourself to your local psychologist for help. You need it.*

If you wish to keep track of how you are doing, you can chart your "leftovers" and see if you are improving (see Leftovers Record.) Since leftovers sometimes end up "trashed" through spoilage or disinterest, that too can be charted. The chart is easily used and quite self explanatory. A sample is shown below. Copies are available in the Appendix.

Table entry codes
 G = went where it was supposed to go. (Positive Feedback.)
 S = spoiled (a real waste)
 E = Went where it was not supposed to go ("I ate the whole thing"!!).
 T = Trashed after stored to avoid eating it.

| Item | Quantity | Outcome |
|------|----------|---------|
| Ardvaark | About ½ pound | S (no one would eat it again) |

## Promises, Resolutions, and Other Potential LIES.

We all tend to lie to ourselves about what we are going to do in our future. We resolve to lose weight, to stop smoking, to stop drinking, to start writing a book, to do a better job, or, my all time favorite: "to turn over a new leaf".

If you have decided to start taking control of your eating behaviour, you are of course at risk of lying to yourself. All the best intentions you may offer yourself are often just not enough to keep you going. Behaviourists have long understood that we need to have some <u>unique</u> way to signal ourselves or remind ourselves of what we are trying to do. I have used a number of such ways with private patients in the past and some seemed pretty silly at the time—but they tended to work. One man carried a small wooden paddle tied to his wrist and on which he kept track of the number of times he did a certain somewhat anti-social behaviour. Another dangled a mechanical counter from their wrist to serve the same purpose. By the time these patients became used to their new attachment, they also had established the habit of being aware of the offending behaviour.

When you undertake to control your eating behaviour, the charting is designed to provide at least part of this unique signal to remind you of what you are trying to do. Any attempt to control your eating behaviour will be so much a part of your day, that you will probably be almost constantly reminded of what you are trying to do for yourself. But if these are not enough, I strongly suggest that you post some of your charts in places such that they will serve to remind you at critical times of exactly what you have resolved to do. Here are some ideas or **"tricks"** to help you along.

1. The refrigerator door is an obvious place for the weight chart. But placing it so that it overlaps the handle makes it especially effective.

2. The place where you keep the "shopping list" is an excellent place for the caloric intake chart—and place it so that it is on top of the shopping list.

3. The activity chart could be placed with your outside clothing so that if you go for a walk you will be reminded both on leaving and returning that you should give yourself credit for this activity.

As you think about this idea of "special signals" to remind yourself of what you are trying to accomplish for yourself, other ideas will strike which reflect your own life style and household organization.

So: **Protect yourself from lying**. Promises and resolutions are great starting places, but give yourself a chance at success and truth telling. **Use unique signals to help you get into the habit of thinking about controlling your eating behaviour**.

The tricks above are just a starting place. Can you find some more or some really unique ones for yourself??

# The Kitchen

Many of your food problems start in this room. It is difficult not to snack as you prepare food. It is difficult not to snack as we walk through a kitchen. It is difficult not to be drawn to the sight and smell of food in the kitchen.

Each shelf and counter may hold food. Some is in cans, jars, boxes, or bags, but some is even exposed and ready to pick up and eat. If it is covered, the label entices you, and if it is open, the smell and/or just plain availability tease you. The open candy dish (or closed one for that matter) is an open invitation to lose control and <u>eat</u>!

Even getting a legitimate glass of cold water from the refrigerator puts you in direct contact with food—especially **leftovers**. The entire house is often invaded by tempting odors coming from the kitchen. And finally, many modern homes almost require you to use the kitchen as a pathway through the house or into the house.

## All this must change!

Here are some **TRICKS** you can consider. Remember that your house and kitchen may not be able to accommodate all of these tricks. And once you get the idea of what you are trying to do, you will probably make up some tricks of your own.

1. Keep food out of sight. This means putting all the food away and closing the cabinet doors. "Out of sight; out of mind," does not really work---but out of sight helps!
2. Secure foods. When you put food away, seal packages, tighten the covers, and generally make it more difficult to get to. This will also keep the food in better condition.
3. Try not to smell up the house. Keep food odors as limited as possible. This means venting the cooking area during food preparation if at all possible. Open windows and outside doors and close inside doors leading to other parts of the house.
4. Keep out of the kitchen. Do not use the kitchen as a social center. Prepare food in the kitchen but do not do anything else there. Only the person preparing food should be in the kitchen if the others are also trying to control their eating behaviour.
5. Limit access to the kitchen space as a means to get from

one place to another. In other words, try to limit the "kitchen traffic" (especially yours.)

6. Store food only in the kitchen. Do not store food or leave food anywhere else in the house. Clean out all food "nests" such as the bedroom cookie bowl, living room candy dish, and the family room nuts (take it either way.)

> **NOTE:** Exception! Some snack foods may be on your list of edibles and be legitimate "between meal snacks". Low calorie and bulky snacks may be left around for those moments of greatest need. But, this does not really help you learn to control your eating behaviour (see Snacking and Snack Foods.)

7. Tasting is not snacking and vice versa. Tasting means getting enough flavor to know that the food is well prepared to your taste. *SNACKING is a polite term for EATING.*

8. Prepare only enough. If you start with too much ingredients, then you will have leftovers or you will risk "preparation snacking". If you do snack while preparing, then you really should reduce the amount you serve yourself on your plate or in your bowl for that meal.

9. No leftovers (see the section on Leftovers.) If you know there is more of a good meal sitting in the kitchen, you will be tempted to go for "seconds".

In summary, do not let your kitchen and its food tease you. Start a list of what you can do and then add to it as you use or discover new **TRICKS.** You can feel good about what you are doing for yourself by seeing what progress you have made by what is appearing on that list.

# Remember, you are attempting to change a whole life style!!

# It will take time!!

# Shopping Techniques

There you are, in your favorite supermarket. You are not sure what you need to buy. You have not planned ahead and brought a shopping list. Instead, you are wandering from aisle to shelf and you see and smell all of the offerings. And the store has done all it can do to make every offering an absolute temptation. What happens?

**You buy what you want**
**Not**
**What you need.**

Not only are you likely to buy foods which you probably should not have, you probably will buy too much of each food. And perhaps even worse, you may be enticed into buying snacks. Some of the snacks will probably be eaten before they and you get home. And those snacks may be forgotten when you try to recall your intake for the day (see Intake Charting.)

Let's face it. Grocery shopping for the hungry, weight controlling, weight losing, food loving person is a potential disaster. The temptation is huge, the store is not interested in helping you cut down your buying or consumption, and you are in a buying frame of mind. It seems that all the cards are stacked against you.

So let's start making this dangerous mission of shopping a little less hazardous. Here are the **TRICKS**!

1. <u>Shop right after eating</u>! I know that is not always possible but when it is, at least you will not be producing saliva with every sight and sound of the store's offerings.
2. <u>Plan ahead</u>. Only go to the store when you have a list of what you really need. Literally, do not allow yourself to go into the store unless you have a list ready.
3. <u>Buy only what is on the list</u>. This is important. If you are shopping and convince yourself that you have left something off of the list because there it is attracting your attention, then add it to the list <u>right then</u>. That gives you a moment more to really think about whether this is something you need or something the store has marketed so well that they "got to you". Even better, and <u>only you true compulsives can do this</u>, leave the store, write the item down on your list while in your car, and then return to the store to

make the purchase. Again, much more time to think this through.

4. <u>How much to buy</u>. Beside each item on your list, show how much of the product you need (see <u>Portion Size</u>.) This is a lot of work. You may spend a lot of time reading food charts. At first, try this with only a few items on your list, until you get used to the idea and start making this a new habit. But do a few items for every list so that you do get into that routine or habit. Of course you will quickly find that stores do not carry cans or jars of just the right quantity. But remember, items which the store packages can be requested to fit exactly your needs (see <u>Leftovers</u> for the treatment of any excess.)

5. <u>Where to shop</u>. If you have to eat less and have to eat things which are not your favorites, at least eat the best quality you can find. And get the service you require. If the store will not honor your needs for special quantities, perhaps another store will be happy to have your business.

6. <u>A matter of money</u>. If possible, pay by check or card. Leave the loose change at home or at least in the car. Cash money is an open invitation to pick up something extra just before you leave the store. Make it very difficult to buy "extras".

**NOTE:** Good buys on large quantities cannot be ignored. But if you buy this way, then do so with the purpose of appropriately storing this large quantity. Make sure you have the proper storage materials on hand. Then process the product as soon as you can. The longer it lingers the more the temptation. Doing the processing after eating reduces the chance of snacking but allows the product to be available for over eating during the meal. Take the alternative here which best reduces your risk.

**Charting**. You can compile your list as simply as you see fit. Or you can make it complex by adding the meal for which the item is intended, the number to be served, and the like. At first, I suggest a simple list with the quantity specified for some of the most important items. As you get into the habit of thinking about portion size, you will quite naturally start to specify this for more of the items on your list.

# Food Preparation

If you are the one preparing food for yourself and others, you are always tempted to taste. Tasting however can easily lead to snacking—which equals eating.

During food preparation, you are at risk through temptation. Extra servings prepared and left on the table, leftovers sitting out in the kitchen, snack foods in open containers—these are all hazards. These hazards and some tricks with which to defend yourself are presented in the section on Leftovers.

If you are the one preparing food, there are many things you can do to help. And remember, you can ask someone else to do these for you if they are preparing the food. Here are some **TRICKS** for you.

1. Make servings look as large as possible. A large plate with little spots of food is immediately going to produce a negative effect. "I can't survive on that" will be heard inside your head, by others around you, or from others who are served that way. Instead, use a smaller plate and crowd it by adding appropriate low calorie items (see Snack Foods.)
2. Prepare the food in small "bite size" pieces whenever possible. They take up more space that way and help you take more time to eat the same amount prepared in larger bites. However, do not at the same time destroy the appearance of the food. A good steak looks best intact—not precut; and it takes time to cut it. But short cut beans take more time to eat than long cut ones and appear to have greater volume.
3. Special care must be taken to make a plate look as nice as possible. All the rules of proper plate presentation should be brought to bear. Remember, you are trying to make your limited food menu and volume as appetizing as possible so that eating will be a positive experience and not a negative one. Plate presentation ideas:
   a. Food should have a variety of colors and not look all alike on the plate. A white plate with white potato and celery sticks for bulk does not have a very appetizing appearance.
   b. Food should have different textures. Each plate should have some soft, some chewy, and some crisp

foods whenever possible.

    c. Food should not always be the same temperature on a plate. A cold salad base with fresh, hot-diced chicken on top is much more fun than a cold salad top to bottom.

    d. Spices and herbs are important. These allow the same product to be served in successive meals and still give you a variety of flavors. For example:

        i. add dill, parsley, basil and oil to potatoes before roasting them.

        ii. cinnamon added to sugar can be sprinkled over plain toast.

        iii. mint added to standard lemonade makes a new drink

        iv. Shallots added to margarine changes plain French bread to a special treat.

4. Finally, if you are preparing food, you may wish to make a large quantity for later use. Your garden produce, a good buy at the store, or a windfall of some specialty require this. But do not allow this to contribute to snacking or overeating.  Put the extra away in storage after it is prepared (see Leftovers.)

Preparing your own food has three great benefits. First, you come to appreciate the effort that it takes and you can feel good about doing that work. Second, when you properly store the leftovers, you can feel good about having "done the right thing". Third, when you eat the food, you again get an appreciation for the work that went into it.

If you wish to, you can chart your success at food preparation on the Master Chart in the Appendix. Seeing how well you are doing is also a way to give yourself Rule Number One by feeling good.

# Intake Charting

If you are truly serious about changing your eating behaviour, in addition to the many "tricks" offered throughout many of the sections of this manual, you will need some way to measure your intake of food. But quantity is not enough. You will need an accurate way to measure intake and an accurate way to decide what you should and should not eat.

To determine what you should and should not eat, you should refer to the section on Food Values.

To determine how many calories you should take in, you should refer to the sections on Goal Setting for Caloric Intake and Food Values.

To determine how much you should eat of any given item, you should refer to the section on Portion Size.

With this information, you can start to do your intake charting.

"Did I eat two or three pieces of toast for breakfast"? We do tend to forget what we have eaten. Especially it is easy to forget how much we have eaten of any one thing. And many times we take (or even sneak) a snack and tell ourselves that it "probably had very few calories anyway" (see Snacking.) You need some way to keep track of your intake from day to day and even during the day. It is especially important to you while you are just learning the caloric values of various foods. The best thing to keep track of is the caloric value of what you are eating. And it is not that difficult. The best time to do the charting is immediately after eating—and that is sometimes harder to do. But do it if at all possible.

There is a chart for you to fill out in the Appendix, and a brief sample of that chart below. Each day you merely list the foods you ate, the caloric value of what you ate, and then the cumulative number of calories for that day. If you wish to, you may also start your chart with the total number of calories which you are allowing yourself each day. Then as you accumulate calories, you can see how you did for each day.

| Date | Food item | # of Calories | Cumulative Calories | Allowable calories |
|------|-----------|---------------|---------------------|--------------------|
| 2/17 | bread | 120 | 120 | 1200 |
| | Cereal | 180 | 300 | |
| | Banana | 114 | 414 | |

**Etc.**

(you might also note that in this example you are about one-third of the way through your total intake allowed for the day.)

**NOTE:** This charting and searching for food values will probably help your shopping effectiveness as well. As you learn the nutritional and caloric values of various foods, you will start buying more of the foods which are appropriate for you. It will make you feel good to see that you stayed within your calorie limit (Rule Number One.)

You will find many uses for your chart. You can see your day's progress in the caloric sense. Are you getting the calories when you need them? Or are you sleeping your calories away? Are you eating your calorie limit so early in the day that you must overdo by evening or go to bed very hungry? You can learn a lot from charting. You may want to chart for only a week or so each month. As you do it more, you will find that it becomes a natural part of your life (habit) and you will be surprised what it may teach you about your eating habits.

Do not forget that having someone help you chart and/or look up nutritional information is a great way to have Rules Number One and Three come into play (see Support People and OTHERS.)

**FINALLY, JUST IN CASE YOU DO NOT WANT TO SPEND TIME WITH FORMAL CHARTING, KEEPING A DIARY OF WHAT YOU HAVE EATEN EACH DAY CAN ACT AS A REMINDER. THIS IS A FORM OF INFORMAL FEEDBACK. YOU MIGHT BE SURPRISED TO FIND THAT YOU ARE ACTUALLY TAKING IN MORE THAN YOU THOUGHT. SEE CHAPTER 8 ON "SNACKING".**

# Celebrations, Sprees, and Socials

It is hard enough to control old (bad) eating habits in normal circumstances. But when you are "out on the town", or having guests in for dinner, or at some other social function, it can be devastatingly hard to keep from snacking or over eating. The temptation can be immense. The social pressure can be very strong. And your favorite calories are usually all laid out before you in a most tantalizing manner. Worse, you may be the one preparing this display of hazardous materials.

What can you do?

I would never recommend that you avoid these otherwise normal social events. Holiday celebrations are important as are many social events where food is a focus or at least plentiful and teasing. Dieting and taking control of your eating should not make a recluse or socially isolated person out of you.

You must learn how to attend these "calorie dates" and still enjoy them without grieving over the loss of snacking or outright eating. Here are some **TRICKS** to try.

**When you are away from your own home:**

1. Keep something in your hands. If your hands are empty, it is easy to pick up food. A purse, small note pad and pen, a piece of clothing which you "may need" or anything else which can keep your hands busy and therefore unable to reach for food serves as a good "block".
2. You can amost always bring your own food with you. You may mildly upset your host the first time, but if you keep it up, you may even get their cooperation in the future. Most true friends will not be offended by your efforts to help yourself.
3. Try to locate yourself away from food—especially if you are at a party where there is a central table of food. Of course if the party is catered and/or served, you may find that the food is brought to you no matter where you place yourself. One way to handle this situation is to ask the server to skip you in the future, "because I am trying to control my eating".
4. Eat something before you go to a food event. Prepare some stomach fillers that are appropriate (see <u>Snack</u>

Foods.) Even if you do not take these with you, you will be less likely to be drawn to the food table because you will feel less hungry.

5. Try to select friends at these parties or celebrations who are supportive of your efforts to control your eating. The idea of having others around you who are understanding and supportive is a good one. They can make you feel good about what you are doing, especially when you control yourself right in front of them. They probably offer you the opportunity of Rules Number One and Three.

**When you are the host and cook:**

1. This is really no different from preparing your own meals. If you are doing any food preparation, then you must be careful to follow the normal rules for <u>Food Preparation</u>. If you are just "hanging around" the food preparation, then perhaps you should go somewhere else.

2. With a lot of luck, you can get a friend to do the food preparation for you. Do not forget to make them understand the need for the proper treatment of <u>Leftovers</u>.

3. If you are the one preparing the food, remember that you can prepare something special for yourself if what you are serving the others is not in your program. They will understand and if they are really good friends, they will often make you feel good by saying how well you are doing (Rules Number One and Three again.)

We are almost all social animals. **Do not deny yourself the company of others or the opportunity to celebrate.**

**But be careful and look after your needs.**

# Support People and OTHERS

For most of you, controlling your eating behaviour would be made much easier if you lived by yourself, cooked only for yourself, ate out by yourself, and otherwise avoided the hazards which others may represent. But in reality, you probably will have to deal with many others. These others can be very positive and helpful, or very negative and hurtful.

Let's look at some typical problem situations:

Case 1. "Mom, I'm hungry. There's nothing in the frig, cookie jar, cabinets or anywhere else around here since you started that stupid diet". Somehow you are going to have to meet this child's need for more food— especially snacks and especially if the child is very active. At the same time, you must protect yourself from the temptation that having all those foods around is going to create. Here are some **TRICKS**.

1. Locate the child's snack food in their own environment.
2. Label the child's snack food (see Leftovers.)
3. Have the child prepare their own snack following the rules of Leftovers after the preparation.
4. Enlist the child's help in Weight Charting. They can fill out the chart with you and see your progress. You get to feel good seeing the progress and the child learns how important this is to you and can also make you feel good by saying so or how well you are doing (Rules Number One and Three.)

Case 2. "I'm not giving up my good dinner for your crazy diet". Well, there really does have to be a trade off between your needs, and the needs of others to not be restricted by your needs. Here again are some **TRICKS**.

1. You can prepare the regular meal for others and serve yourself either separately or just less.
2. Take special care to produce an especially fine meal for the "others". Perhaps a little guilt will make them make you feel good by noting how well you are controlling yourself (Rules Number One and Three.)
3. Assure the "others" that you are making progress and again there is the opportunity to have them make you feel good about yourself and what you are doing.
4. **Finally, substitute "child" for "others" and see all of the tricks for Case 1.**

Case 3. "Aw come on. You can try just one". "One can't hurt you". "You make me feel guilty just watching and not enjoying this with me". "I went to a lot of trouble to make this so please at least have one so you can tell me if I did a good job". Do not fall for these attempts to cause a break in your reality and routine (see <u>Beware the Mini Psychosis</u>.) These "helpful" comments can come from friends and family as they seek their own good feeling via Rules Number One and Three. Here are some possible **TRICKS** and ideas.

1. Be very open and direct with these folks. Tell them you are trying to do something very positive for yourself. Tell them that you feel badly for them that you cannot take what they offer, but that you are firm in your resolve to take appropriate steps in your behaviour control program.

2. Try to help them understand that you would like their support. "I know you are my friend so I know that I can count of you to help me stay on my routine". "I will keep you posted on how I am doing". "You should see all the things I have learned about how to control my eating". This may help divert their attention from their needs to yours.

3. Relieve their guilt by showing them what foods will satisfy your needs and therefore make you happy about yourself. Again you are trying to divert their attention from their needs to being a positive help to yours.

Generally, enlisting others to help you research, make up menus, or even chart your success, is best. They can provide you with that positive feedback which feels so good.

Each of the cases above reflect the initial reactions of those around someone trying to gain control over their eating. This initial reaction usually can be changed if you do not overburden others with your needs at the start. Gradually let them become a part of your program. Helping them understand will most likely result in their providing you with those all important Rules Number One and Three happenings.

# Eating Style

As mentioned in the introduction, the big three of eating problems are: eating too fast, eating too much, and eating too often. Eating too often is usually a matter of snacking and is dealt with in the <u>Snacking</u> section of the manual. Eating too much can be the result of eating too fast or the result of poor proportion planning and food preparation. Refer to the <u>Shopping Techniques</u> and <u>Food Preparation</u> sections respectively for this information.

Eating too fast is a significant problem. Often the fast eater is the first one through the meal. You end up watching others eat. And it is very difficult to watch others eat when you still feel hungry. And why do you still feel hungry? Because you probably ate so fast that your body has not yet recognized that you are full. It has not yet had time to send that signal to you that you have taken in enough. The result is of course that you begin to eat again.

You may tell yourself that you are eating again because you are still hungry, but we (you and I) know that that is probably not true. You may tell yourself that it is not polite to not join the others and just sit there and watch them. But the truth is, it was not polite of you to eat so fast that you ended up finished well ahead of the pack.

Here is a **TRICK** for you. To slow your pace, just set your fork or spoon down between bites. And since there is not another bite headed immediately to your mouth, you can concentrate on the mouthful you have. Both the act of putting your spoon down and concentrating on the current mouthful will force you to slow down the rate at which you are eating your way through the plate.

The second aspect of eating too fast is that you may be taking very large mouthfuls. Spoonful or forkful does not have to mean "<u>as full as I can get it</u>". Here is another **TRICK** for you. Use small utensils. While there are those socialites which will say that soup must be eaten with a soup spoon, a regular tea spoon may be a much more appropriate size. You will be forced to take many more "spoonfuls" and that will also reduce the rate at which you are eating. Smaller forks also help.

Of course, no "eating style" lesson would be complete without appealing to your sense of the food itself. Savor the food. Savor each bite. Let the flavors run around your mouth and tongue to taste what is in the food. By enjoying these flavors more, you are invoking Rule Number One, and at a good time for Rule Number Three.

## Do Not Just Swallow! Savor!

Yet another **TRICK** to delay the eating rate has to do with what you might do between each bite. Savor it of course. But talking is a very acceptable behavior also (after swallowing of course.) I personally like the Chinese approach to dinner table conversation: talk about the food you are eating and the foods you have had in the past! They generally consider it impolite to talk about anything else. Since you are savoring the mouthful, you will probably be learning more about the food and therefore have more to say about it than you thought.

I have put a Master Chart in the Appendix. This will give you a chance to record a number of aspects of your daily eating. At the end of each meal you may note the time you spent and whether this was too much time, too little, or "ok". You also have space to note that you did or did not "savor", set aside the fork or spoon, or talk. You will be able to see your progress in controlling your behaviour by looking back at earlier days and therefore be able to say to yourself that "I am doing well" or that "I need to work on that more".

# Moods

As a psychologist, I just cannot pass up the opportunity to address this potential problem.

*All of us eat to live, others live to eat.*

All of us need to be careful of our food intake lest we fail to take in the necessary distribution of foods (see <u>Food Values</u>.) But those of you who live for food are at extra risk, that you will take in too much of almost everything. Being a true gourmand, I have faced this risk regularly and know of which I speak.

But those of you who live to eat, and those who are gourmands, are not in the same category of risk as those of you who are "mood eaters".

Most people experience occasional mood swings. Mood swings are perfectly normal and are not necessarily the cause of out of control easting. We go from happy to sad or feeling low to feeling great. These swings usually reflect what is happening around and to us at the time.

However, for a few, these moods are almost always overpowering in their demand that we eat. The old idea that we "eat away our problems" is both true and false. It is true that some eat when they have problems or feel low. But it is false that the problems or low feelings go away with eating. Quite the contrary! The eating usually makes matters worse by making you feel worse about yourself for potentially gaining weight and risking your health.

If you are a mood eater, you may wish to seek some help from your local counselor. There is often a reason that can be addressed and set you free from this problem.

If your moods and mood swings are great and frequent, then I <u>strongly recommend the trip to your counselor</u>. Moods which are so low that you feel you can do nothing to help yourself or that nothing is exciting or even of mild interest to you, are dangerous. Similarly, moods which are so high that you feel totally invulnerable, totally capable, and without control over such things as spending or engaging in excessive behaviours of almost every kind, are equally dangerous.

## Beware The Mini Psychosis

When you hear yourself say "Oh I can eat that, I'll just starve a little later on (sometime)", you are at the very least bordering upon a very brief but very real state of <u>MINI PSYCHOSIS</u>. Briefly, psychosis is the loss of touch with reality. A mini psychosis is a very brief event. It usually occurs when we <u>lie</u> to ourselves about something which we know is not true. In other words, when we start believing our lies.

### Let me tell you a story:

In about 1965 I finally stopped smoking after many years of polluting my environment and that of many others. In about 1974, a psychiatrist and I spent a day working together and decided to reward ourselves by having a "fine dining" experience. As the meal came to a close and the Brandy was served, the following conversation occurred.

Psychiatrist: (while pulling a pair of huge and wonderful Cuban cigars from his breast pocket) "Dick, this meal and the Brandy deserve a cigar. Here, I brought these especially for this occasion."
Dick: "Hey, I don't smoke. I had to quit because I inhale every breath of smoke. Even cigars and pipe smoke. I just had to quit."
Psychiatrist: (about two minutes later, after lighting and dipping the cigar into the Brandy) "This cigar is just perfect. What a flavor and aroma. I'm sorry you can't enjoy one with me."
Dick: (and here comes the break from reality) "Oh, I could have just one. Just one couldn't hurt me. I won't have a chance to have another like that again for quite a while.  And I can certainly keep from having anything else to smoke."

So I did. The next day I thought again that I could just have one cigar for lunch—then two during the evening—then—and then—. The mini psychosis was finally recognized for what it was as I shifted to cigarettes in order to protect my health from the cigar smoke. I was "hooked" again. I was unable to stop smoking for about six years.

Beware the mini psychosis. It is a sneaky event. It can attack at any time. When you hear yourself start to lie about your reality:

# STOP ! ! !

(if you can)

# Where to Eat

Food spread all over the house just makes for temptation. It also makes it easier to take a quick snack. Similarly, eating food at many locations in the house strengthens your habit of eating anywhere you like. Finally, eating in many locations of the house allows you to associate food with all those places and the activities which you do in those places. Each of these locations is going to work against you by reminding you that food has been available in them. Worse, many of these places will be associated with "junk food" or "snacks".

Here are some guidelines or "**TRICKS**".

1. Try to eat all your meals in one place. This then associates eating with that place alone and starts to break the habit of casual eating elsewhere in the house.
2. Select a place in which as little else goes on as possible.
    a. Some homes have dining rooms which are separate <u>rooms</u>. These are especially good places to eat from this point of view. But do not let them become a sewing table, study desk, or model airplane bench during "off hours". Use only for dining if at all possible.
    b. Many modern houses have an eating area which is part of the kitchen. If this is your situation, then make this area as separate from the kitchen as possible. Use a divider or hanging plants to separate the two areas. **TRICK**! Turn off the kitchen lights and turn on the light over or around the eating area. This may also help to separate the two areas.
    c. Finally, clear the table completely. All reminders that the table is for eating should disappear. The place mats, table cloth, special center piece, the silverware, and dishes all are reminders of "eating" and can make you feel hungry at times when you are not scheduled to eat. Then if the table is used for something else, at least it is not so closely associated with eating.

The whole idea here is to try to break up the association between food and all activities and places in the house, so that eating is only thought of in your "eating place".

# Activity Charting

Charting your activity level is something which, like all other charting, you should start doing slowly until you "get into the habit". It is really very easy and there are charts in the Appendix. Merely enter the caloric value of the activities you had for the day. You will find these in the Caloric Output Charts in the Appendix. Add up the calories and you have the number for your day's efforts.

Since it is not always easy to recall all of the activities you may do during a day, as you get used to charting, you may find that charting at lunch as well as at the end of the day will be very helpful.

Here is a sample of an Activity Chart.

(Enter the number of calories used during each activity)

| Date | | | | | | | | | | | | | | | | | | | | | | | | | |
|---|---|---|---|---|---|---|---|---|---|---|---|---|---|---|---|---|---|---|---|---|---|---|---|---|---|
| Activity | | | | | | | | | | | | | | | | | | | | | | | | | |
| Swimming* | | | | | | | | | | | | | | | | | | | | | | | | | |
| Walking* | | | | | | | | | | | | | | | | | | | | | | | | | |
| Standing at counter* | | | | | | | | | | | | | | | | | | | | | | | | | |
| Reading* | | | | | | | | | | | | | | | | | | | | | | | | | |
| Other* | | | | | | | | | | | | | | | | | | | | | | | | | |

*Note that when you start this kind of charting, you will find that many of your types of activity remain the same from day to day. Put these first on your chart. The less frequently used activities will gradually lengthen the list and you will finally use "other" for very rare activities.

Note also that for each of these activities the number of calories to enter in the box for that date depends on how long you did the activity. So you must look up in the Caloric Output Chart in the Appendix and determine how much credit to give yourself based upon how long you were at the activity.

# Weight Chart

| Weight | | | | | | | | | | | | | | | | | | | | | | | | | | |
|---|---|---|---|---|---|---|---|---|---|---|---|---|---|---|---|---|---|---|---|---|---|---|---|---|---|---|

**Days**

# Weight Chart

| Weight | | | | | | | | | | | | | | | | | | | | | | | | | |
|---|---|---|---|---|---|---|---|---|---|---|---|---|---|---|---|---|---|---|---|---|---|---|---|---|---|

**Days**

# Weight Chart

| Weight | | | | | | | | | | | | | | | | | | | | | | | | | | | | | | | | |
|---|---|---|---|---|---|---|---|---|---|---|---|---|---|---|---|---|---|---|---|---|---|---|---|---|---|---|---|---|---|---|---|---|

**Days**

# Weight Chart

| Weight | | | | | | | | | | | | | | | | | | | | | | | | | | | | | | | | | | | | | | | | | | | |
|---|---|---|---|---|---|---|---|---|---|---|---|---|---|---|---|---|---|---|---|---|---|---|---|---|---|---|---|---|---|---|---|---|---|---|---|---|---|---|---|---|---|---|---|---|
| | | | | | | | | | | | | | | | | | | | | | | | | | | | | | | | | | | | | | | | | | | | | |

**Days**

# Activity Chart

(Enter the number of calories used during each activity)

| Date | | | | | | | | | | | | | | | | | | | | | | | |
|------|--|--|--|--|--|--|--|--|--|--|--|--|--|--|--|--|--|--|--|--|--|--|--|
| Activity | | | | | | | | | | | | | | | | | | | | | | | |
| | | | | | | | | | | | | | | | | | | | | | | | |
| | | | | | | | | | | | | | | | | | | | | | | | |
| | | | | | | | | | | | | | | | | | | | | | | | |
| | | | | | | | | | | | | | | | | | | | | | | | |
| | | | | | | | | | | | | | | | | | | | | | | | |
| | | | | | | | | | | | | | | | | | | | | | | | |
| | | | | | | | | | | | | | | | | | | | | | | | |
| | | | | | | | | | | | | | | | | | | | | | | | |
| | | | | | | | | | | | | | | | | | | | | | | | |
| | | | | | | | | | | | | | | | | | | | | | | | |
| | | | | | | | | | | | | | | | | | | | | | | | |

# Activity Chart

(Enter the number of calories used during each activity)

| Date | | | | | | | | | | | | | | | | | | | | | | | | | | | | | | | | |
|------|---|---|---|---|---|---|---|---|---|---|---|---|---|---|---|---|---|---|---|---|---|---|---|---|---|---|---|---|---|---|---|---|---|
| Activity | | | | | | | | | | | | | | | | | | | | | | | | | | | | | | | | | |
| | | | | | | | | | | | | | | | | | | | | | | | | | | | | | | | | | |
| | | | | | | | | | | | | | | | | | | | | | | | | | | | | | | | | | |
| | | | | | | | | | | | | | | | | | | | | | | | | | | | | | | | | | |
| | | | | | | | | | | | | | | | | | | | | | | | | | | | | | | | | | |
| | | | | | | | | | | | | | | | | | | | | | | | | | | | | | | | | | |
| | | | | | | | | | | | | | | | | | | | | | | | | | | | | | | | | | |
| | | | | | | | | | | | | | | | | | | | | | | | | | | | | | | | | | |
| | | | | | | | | | | | | | | | | | | | | | | | | | | | | | | | | | |
| | | | | | | | | | | | | | | | | | | | | | | | | | | | | | | | | | |
| | | | | | | | | | | | | | | | | | | | | | | | | | | | | | | | | | |
| | | | | | | | | | | | | | | | | | | | | | | | | | | | | | | | | | |
| | | | | | | | | | | | | | | | | | | | | | | | | | | | | | | | | | |
| | | | | | | | | | | | | | | | | | | | | | | | | | | | | | | | | | |
| | | | | | | | | | | | | | | | | | | | | | | | | | | | | | | | | | |
| | | | | | | | | | | | | | | | | | | | | | | | | | | | | | | | | | |
| | | | | | | | | | | | | | | | | | | | | | | | | | | | | | | | | | |
| | | | | | | | | | | | | | | | | | | | | | | | | | | | | | | | | | |
| | | | | | | | | | | | | | | | | | | | | | | | | | | | | | | | | | |
| | | | | | | | | | | | | | | | | | | | | | | | | | | | | | | | | | |
| | | | | | | | | | | | | | | | | | | | | | | | | | | | | | | | | | |
| | | | | | | | | | | | | | | | | | | | | | | | | | | | | | | | | | |
| | | | | | | | | | | | | | | | | | | | | | | | | | | | | | | | | | |
| | | | | | | | | | | | | | | | | | | | | | | | | | | | | | | | | | |

# Activity Chart

(Enter the number of calories used during each activity)

| Date | | | | | | | | | | | | | | | | | | | | | | | | | | | | |
|------|---|---|---|---|---|---|---|---|---|---|---|---|---|---|---|---|---|---|---|---|---|---|---|---|---|---|---|---|---|
| Activity | | | | | | | | | | | | | | | | | | | | | | | | | | | | |
| | | | | | | | | | | | | | | | | | | | | | | | | | | | | | |
| | | | | | | | | | | | | | | | | | | | | | | | | | | | | | |
| | | | | | | | | | | | | | | | | | | | | | | | | | | | | | |
| | | | | | | | | | | | | | | | | | | | | | | | | | | | | | |
| | | | | | | | | | | | | | | | | | | | | | | | | | | | | | |
| | | | | | | | | | | | | | | | | | | | | | | | | | | | | | |
| | | | | | | | | | | | | | | | | | | | | | | | | | | | | | |
| | | | | | | | | | | | | | | | | | | | | | | | | | | | | | |

# Master Chart

(score time, yes or no, number, good{G} or bad{B})

Dates

| | | | | | | | | | | | | | | | | | | | | | | |
|---|---|---|---|---|---|---|---|---|---|---|---|---|---|---|---|---|---|---|---|---|---|---|
| Eating Style | | | | | | | | | | | | | | | | | | | | | | |
|    Did you savor the food? | | | | | | | | | | | | | | | | | | | | | | |
|    Did you take enough time? | | | | | | | | | | | | | | | | | | | | | | |
|    Did you talk between bites? | | | | | | | | | | | | | | | | | | | | | | |
|    Did you pause between bites? | | | | | | | | | | | | | | | | | | | | | | |
| Food Preparation | | | | | | | | | | | | | | | | | | | | | | |
|    Were your portions good? | | | | | | | | | | | | | | | | | | | | | | |
|    Did you snack? | | | | | | | | | | | | | | | | | | | | | | |
|    Did the plates/food look good? | | | | | | | | | | | | | | | | | | | | | | |
|    Did you care for leftovers? | | | | | | | | | | | | | | | | | | | | | | |
| Snacks | | | | | | | | | | | | | | | | | | | | | | |
|    When did you snack? | | | | | | | | | | | | | | | | | | | | | | |
|    Where did you snack? | | | | | | | | | | | | | | | | | | | | | | |
|    Was the snack appropriate? | | | | | | | | | | | | | | | | | | | | | | |
|    Did you turn down a snack? | | | | | | | | | | | | | | | | | | | | | | |

# Master Chart

(score time, yes or no, number, good{G} or bad{B})

Dates

| | | | | | | | | | | | | | | | | | | | | | | |
|---|---|---|---|---|---|---|---|---|---|---|---|---|---|---|---|---|---|---|---|---|---|---|
| **Eating Style** | | | | | | | | | | | | | | | | | | | | | | |
| Did you savor the food? | | | | | | | | | | | | | | | | | | | | | | |
| Did you take enough time? | | | | | | | | | | | | | | | | | | | | | | |
| Did you talk between bites? | | | | | | | | | | | | | | | | | | | | | | |
| Did you pause between bites? | | | | | | | | | | | | | | | | | | | | | | |
| **Food Preparation** | | | | | | | | | | | | | | | | | | | | | | |
| Were your portions good? | | | | | | | | | | | | | | | | | | | | | | |
| Did you snack? | | | | | | | | | | | | | | | | | | | | | | |
| Did the plates/food look good? | | | | | | | | | | | | | | | | | | | | | | |
| Did you care for leftovers? | | | | | | | | | | | | | | | | | | | | | | |
| **Snacks** | | | | | | | | | | | | | | | | | | | | | | |
| When did you snack? | | | | | | | | | | | | | | | | | | | | | | |
| Where did you snack? | | | | | | | | | | | | | | | | | | | | | | |
| Was the snack appropriate? | | | | | | | | | | | | | | | | | | | | | | |
| Did you turn down a snack? | | | | | | | | | | | | | | | | | | | | | | |

# Intake Chart

| | Food Item | # of Calories | Cumulative Calories | Allowable Calories |
|---|---|---|---|---|
| | | | | |
| | | | | |
| | | | | |
| | | | | |
| | | | | |
| | | | | |
| | | | | |
| | | | | |
| | | | | |
| | | | | |
| | | | | |
| | | | | |
| | | | | |
| | | | | |
| | | | | |
| | | | | |
| | | | | |
| | | | | |
| | | | | |
| | | | | |
| | | | | |
| | | | | |
| | | | | |
| | | | | |

# Intake Chart

| | Food Item | # of Calories | Cumulative Calories | Allowable Calories |
|---|---|---|---|---|
| | | | | |
| | | | | |
| | | | | |
| | | | | |
| | | | | |
| | | | | |
| | | | | |
| | | | | |
| | | | | |
| | | | | |
| | | | | |
| | | | | |
| | | | | |
| | | | | |
| | | | | |
| | | | | |
| | | | | |
| | | | | |
| | | | | |
| | | | | |
| | | | | |
| | | | | |
| | | | | |
| | | | | |

# Leftover Record

Table entry codes
- G = Went where it was supposed to go.
- S = Spoiled (a real waste).
- E = Went where it was not supposed to go (I ate the whole thing).
- T = Trashed after stored to avoid eating it.

| Item | Quantity | Outcome |
| --- | --- | --- |
| | | |
| | | |
| | | |
| | | |
| | | |
| | | |
| | | |
| | | |
| | | |
| | | |
| | | |
| | | |
| | | |
| | | |
| | | |
| | | |
| | | |
| | | |
| | | |
| | | |
| | | |
| | | |
| | | |
| | | |
| | | |
| | | |
| | | |
| | | |

# Appendix C

# Approximate Caloric Expenditure Per Minute for Various Physical Activities*

Permission granted by the McGraw-Hill Companies to reproduce this Appendix from Wiilliams, M. Nutrition For Fitness and Sport, 1988. Wm C Brown Publishers, Dubuque, Iowa

**Body weight**

| | | KG | 45 | 48 | 50 | 52 | 55 | 57 | 59 | 61 | 64 | 66 | 68 | 70 |
|---|---|---|---|---|---|---|---|---|---|---|---|---|---|---|
| | | Pounds | 100 | 105 | 110 | 115 | 120 | 125 | 130 | 135 | 140 | 145 | 150 | 155 |

*Sedentary activities*

| | 45 | 48 | 50 | 52 | 55 | 57 | 59 | 61 | 64 | 66 | 68 | 70 |
|---|---|---|---|---|---|---|---|---|---|---|---|---|
| Lying quietly | .99 | 1.0 | 1.1 | 1.1 | 1.2 | 1.3 | 1.3 | 1.4 | 1.4 | 1.5 | 1.5 | 1.5 |
| Sitting and writing, card playing, etc. | 1.2 | 1.3 | 1.4 | 1.5 | 1.5 | 1.6 | 1.7 | 1.7 | 1.8 | 1.8 | 1.9 | 2.0 |
| Standing with light work, cleaning, etc. | 2.7 | 2.9 | 3.0 | 3.1 | 3.3 | 3.4 | 3.5 | 3.7 | 3.8 | 3.9 | 4.1 | 4.2 |

*Physical activities*

| | 45 | 48 | 50 | 52 | 55 | 57 | 59 | 61 | 64 | 66 | 68 | 70 |
|---|---|---|---|---|---|---|---|---|---|---|---|---|
| Archery | 3.1 | 3.3 | 3.5 | 3.6 | 3.8 | 4.0 | 4.1 | 4.3 | 4.5 | 4.6 | 4.8 | 4.9 |
| Badminton | | | | | | | | | | | | |
|   Recreational singles | 3.6 | 3.8 | 4.0 | 4.2 | 4.4 | 4.6 | 4.7 | 4.9 | 5.1 | 5.3 | 5.4 | 5.6 |
|   Social doubles | 2.7 | 2.9 | 3.0 | 3.1 | 3.3 | 3.4 | 3.5 | 3.7 | 3.8 | 3.9 | 4.1 | 4.2 |
|   Competitive | 5.9 | 6.1 | 6.4 | 6.7 | 7.0 | 7.3 | 7.6 | 7.9 | 8.2 | 8.5 | 8.8 | 9.1 |
| Baseball | | | | | | | | | | | | |
|   Player | 3.1 | 3.3 | 3.4 | 3.6 | 3.8 | 4.0 | 4.1 | 4.3 | 4.4 | 4.5 | 4.7 | 4.8 |
|   Pitcher | 3.9 | 4.1 | 4.3 | 4.5 | 4.7 | 4.9 | 5.1 | 5.3 | 5.5 | 5.7 | 5.9 | 6.0 |
| Basketball | | | | | | | | | | | | |
|   Half court | 3.0 | 3.1 | 3.3 | 3.5 | 3.6 | 3.8 | 3.9 | 4.1 | 4.2 | 4.4 | 4.5 | 4.7 |
|   Recreational | 4.9 | 5.2 | 5.5 | 5.7 | 6.0 | 6.2 | 6.5 | 6.7 | 7.0 | 7.2 | 7.5 | 7.7 |
|   Vigorous competition | 6.5 | 6.8 | 7.2 | 7.5 | 7.8 | 8.2 | 8.5 | 8.8 | 9.2 | 9.5 | 9.9 | 10.2 |

Bicycling, level

| (mph) | (min/mile) | 45 | 48 | 50 | 52 | 55 | 57 | 59 | 61 | 64 | 66 | 68 | 70 |
|---|---|---|---|---|---|---|---|---|---|---|---|---|---|
| 5 | 12:00 | 1.9 | 2.0 | 2.1 | 2.2 | 2.3 | 2.4 | 2.5 | 2.6 | 2.7 | 2.8 | 2.9 | 3.0 |
| 10 | 6:00 | 4.2 | 4.4 | 4.6 | 4.8 | 5.1 | 5.3 | 5.5 | 5.7 | 5.9 | 6.1 | 6.4 | 6.6 |
| 15 | 4:00 | 7.3 | 7.6 | 8.0 | 8.4 | 8.7 | 9.1 | 9.5 | 9.8 | 10.0 | 10.5 | 10.9 | 11.3 |
| 20 | 3:00 | 10.7 | 11.2 | 11.7 | 12.3 | 12.8 | 13.3 | 13.9 | 14.4 | 14.9 | 15.5 | 16.0 | 16.5 |
| Bowling | | 2.7 | 2.8 | 3.0 | 3.1 | 3.3 | 3.4 | 3.5 | 3.7 | 3.8 | 3.9 | 4.1 | 4.2 |

*Note: The energy cost, in Calories, will vary for different physical activities in a given individual depending on various factors. For example, the caloric cost of bicycling will vary depending on the type of bicycle, going uphill or downhill, and wind resistance. Walking with hand weights or ankle weights will increase energy output. Thus, the values expressed here are approximations and may be increased or decreased depending upon factors that influence energy cost.

| 73 | 75 | 77 | 80 | 82 | 84 | 86 | 89 | 91 | 93 | 95 | 98 | 100 |
|----|----|----|----|----|----|----|----|----|----|----|----|-----|
| 160 | 165 | 170 | 175 | 180 | 185 | 190 | 195 | 200 | 205 | 210 | 215 | 220 |
| 1.6 | 1.6 | 1.7 | 1.7 | 1.8 | 1.8 | 1.9 | 1.9 | 2.0 | 2.0 | 2.1 | 2.1 | 2.2 |
| 2.0 | 2.1 | 2.2 | 2.2 | 2.3 | 2.4 | 2.4 | 2.5 | 2.5 | 2.6 | 2.7 | 2.7 | 2.8 |
| 4.4 | 4.5 | 4.6 | 4.8 | 4.9 | 5.0 | 5.2 | 5.3 | 5.4 | 5.6 | 5.7 | 5.9 | 6.0 |
| 5.1 | 5.3 | 5.4 | 5.6 | 5.7 | 5.9 | 6.0 | 6.2 | 6.4 | 6.5 | 6.7 | 6.9 | 7.0 |
| 5.8 | 6.0 | 6.2 | 6.4 | 6.6 | 6.7 | 6.9 | 7.1 | 7.3 | 7.4 | 7.6 | 7.8 | 8.0 |
| 4.4 | 4.5 | 4.6 | 4.8 | 4.9 | 5.0 | 5.2 | 5.3 | 5.4 | 5.6 | 5.7 | 5.9 | 6.0 |
| 9.4 | 9.7 | 10.0 | 10.3 | 10.6 | 10.9 | 11.2 | 11.5 | 11.8 | 12.1 | 12.4 | 12.7 | 13.0 |
| 5.0 | 5.2 | 5.3 | 5.5 | 5.6 | 5.8 | 5.9 | 6.1 | 6.3 | 6.4 | 6.6 | 6.8 | 6.9 |
| 6.3 | 6.5 | 6.7 | 6.9 | 7.1 | 7.3 | 7.4 | 7.7 | 7.9 | 8.0 | 8.2 | 8.5 | 8.6 |
| 4.8 | 5.0 | 5.1 | 5.3 | 5.4 | 5.6 | 5.7 | 5.9 | 6.0 | 6.2 | 6.4 | 6.5 | 6.7 |
| 8.0 | 8.2 | 8.5 | 8.7 | 9.0 | 9.2 | 9.5 | 9.7 | 10.0 | 10.2 | 10.5 | 10.7 | 11.0 |
| 10.5 | 10.9 | 11.2 | 11.5 | 11.9 | 12.2 | 12.5 | 12.9 | 13.2 | 13.5 | 13.8 | 14.2 | 14.5 |
| 3.1 | 3.2 | 3.3 | 3.4 | 3.5 | 3.6 | 3.7 | 3.8 | 3.9 | 4.0 | 4.1 | 4.2 | 4.3 |
| 6.8 | 7.0 | 7.2 | 7.4 | 7.6 | 7.9 | 8.1 | 8.3 | 8.5 | 8.7 | 8.9 | 9.1 | 9.4 |
| 11.6 | 12.0 | 12.4 | 12.7 | 13.1 | 13.4 | 13.8 | 14.2 | 14.5 | 14.9 | 15.3 | 15.6 | 16.0 |
| 17.1 | 17.6 | 18.1 | 18.7 | 19.2 | 19.7 | 20.3 | 20.8 | 21.3 | 21.9 | 22.4 | 22.9 | 23.5 |
| 4.4 | 4.5 | 4.6 | 4.8 | 4.9 | 5.0 | 5.2 | 5.3 | 5.5 | 5.6 | 5.7 | 5.9 | 6.0 |

**Body weight**

| | KG | 45 | 48 | 50 | 52 | 55 | 57 | 59 | 61 | 64 | 66 | 68 | 70 |
|---|---|---|---|---|---|---|---|---|---|---|---|---|---|
| | Pounds | 100 | 105 | 110 | 115 | 120 | 125 | 130 | 135 | 140 | 145 | 150 | 155 |
| Calisthenics | | | | | | | | | | | | | |
| Light type | | 3.4 | 3.6 | 3.8 | 4.0 | 4.1 | 4.3 | 4.5 | 4.7 | 4.8 | 5.0 | 5.2 | 5.4 |
| Timed vigorous | | 9.7 | 10.1 | 10.6 | 11.1 | 11.6 | 12.1 | 12.6 | 13.1 | 13.6 | 14.1 | 14.6 | 15.1 |
| Canoeing | | | | | | | | | | | | | |
| (mph) | (min/mile) | | | | | | | | | | | | |
| 2.5 | 24 | 1.9 | 2.0 | 2.1 | 2.2 | 2.3 | 2.4 | 2.5 | 2.6 | 2.7 | 2.8 | 2.9 | 3.0 |
| 4.0 | 15 | 4.4 | 4.6 | 4.9 | 5.1 | 5.3 | 5.5 | 5.8 | 6.0 | 6.2 | 6.4 | 6.7 | 6.9 |
| 5.0 | 12 | 5.7 | 6.0 | 6.3 | 6.6 | 6.9 | 7.2 | 7.5 | 7.8 | 8.1 | 8.4 | 8.7 | 9.0 |
| Dancing | | | | | | | | | | | | | |
| Moderately (waltz) | | 3.1 | 3.3 | 3.5 | 3.6 | 3.8 | 4.0 | 4.1 | 4.3 | 4.5 | 4.6 | 4.8 | 4.9 |
| Active (square, disco) | | 4.5 | 4.7 | 5.0 | 5.2 | 5.4 | 5.6 | 5.9 | 6.1 | 6.3 | 6.6 | 6.8 | 7.0 |
| Aerobic (vigorously) | | 6.0 | 6.3 | 6.7 | 7.0 | 7.3 | 7.6 | 7.9 | 8.2 | 8.5 | 8.8 | 9.1 | 9.4 |
| Fencing | | | | | | | | | | | | | |
| Moderately | | 3.3 | 3.5 | 3.6 | 3.8 | 4.0 | 4.1 | 4.3 | 4.5 | 4.6 | 4.8 | 5.0 | 5.2 |
| Vigorously | | 6.6 | 7.0 | 7.3 | 7.7 | 8.0 | 8.3 | 8.7 | 9.0 | 9.4 | 9.7 | 10.0 | 10.4 |
| Field hockey | | 5.0 | 6.3 | 6.7 | 7.0 | 7.3 | 7.6 | 7.9 | 8.2 | 8.5 | 8.8 | 9.1 | 9.4 |
| Football | | | | | | | | | | | | | |
| Moderate | | 3.3 | 3.5 | 3.6 | 3.8 | 4.0 | 4.1 | 4.3 | 4.5 | 4.6 | 4.8 | 5.0 | 5.2 |
| Touch, vigorous | | 5.5 | 5.8 | 6.1 | 6.4 | 6.6 | 6.9 | 7.2 | 7.5 | 7.8 | 8.0 | 8.3 | 8.6 |
| Golf | | | | | | | | | | | | | |
| 2-some (carry clubs) | | 3.6 | 3.8 | 4.0 | 4.2 | 4.4 | 4.6 | 4.7 | 4.9 | 5.1 | 5.3 | 5.4 | 5.6 |
| 4-some (carry clubs) | | 2.7 | 2.9 | 3.0 | 3.1 | 3.3 | 3.4 | 3.5 | 3.7 | 3.8 | 3.9 | 4.1 | 4.2 |
| Power-cart | | 1.9 | 2.0 | 2.1 | 2.2 | 2.3 | 2.4 | 2.5 | 2.6 | 2.7 | 2.8 | 2.9 | 3.0 |
| Handball | | | | | | | | | | | | | |
| Moderate | | 6.5 | 6.8 | 7.2 | 7.5 | 7.8 | 8.2 | 8.5 | 8.8 | 9.2 | 9.5 | 9.9 | 10.2 |
| Competitive | | 7.7 | 8.0 | 8.4 | 8.8 | 9.2 | 9.6 | 10.0 | 10.4 | 10.8 | 11.1 | 11.5 | 11.9 |
| Hiking, pack (3 mph) | | 4.5 | 4.7 | 5.0 | 5.2 | 5.4 | 5.6 | 5.9 | 6.1 | 6.3 | 6.6 | 6.8 | 7.0 |
| Hocky, ice | | 6.6 | 7.0 | 7.3 | 7.7 | 8.0 | 8.3 | 8.7 | 9.0 | 9.4 | 9.7 | 10.0 | 10.4 |

| 73 | 75 | 77 | 80 | 82 | 84 | 86 | 89 | 91 | 93 | 95 | 98 | 100 |
|---|---|---|---|---|---|---|---|---|---|---|---|---|
| 160 | 165 | 170 | 175 | 180 | 185 | 190 | 195 | 200 | 205 | 210 | 215 | 220 |

| 73 | 75 | 77 | 80 | 82 | 84 | 86 | 89 | 91 | 93 | 95 | 98 | 100 |
|---|---|---|---|---|---|---|---|---|---|---|---|---|
| 5.5 | 5.7 | 5.9 | 6.1 | 6.3 | 6.4 | 6.6 | 6.8 | 7.0 | 7.1 | 7.3 | 7.5 | 7.7 |
| 15.6 | 16.1 | 16.6 | 17.1 | 17.6 | 18.1 | 18.6 | 19.1 | 19.6 | 20.0 | 20.5 | 21.0 | 21.5 |

| 3.1 | 3.2 | 3.3 | 3.4 | 3.5 | 3.6 | 3.7 | 3.8 | 3.9 | 4.0 | 4.1 | 4.2 | 4.3 |
|---|---|---|---|---|---|---|---|---|---|---|---|---|
| 7.1 | 7.4 | 7.6 | 7.8 | 8.0 | 8.2 | 8.5 | 8.7 | 8.9 | 9.1 | 9.4 | 9.6 | 9.8 |
| 9.3 | 9.5 | 9.8 | 10.1 | 10.4 | 10.7 | 11.0 | 11.3 | 11.6 | 11.9 | 12.2 | 12.5 | 12.8 |

| 5.1 | 5.3 | 5.4 | 5.6 | 5.7 | 5.9 | 6.0 | 6.2 | 6.4 | 6.5 | 6.7 | 6.9 | 7.0 |
|---|---|---|---|---|---|---|---|---|---|---|---|---|
| 7.3 | 7.5 | 7.7 | 7.9 | 8.2 | 8.4 | 8.6 | 8.9 | 9.1 | 9.3 | 9.5 | 9.8 | 10.0 |
| 9.7 | 10.0 | 10.3 | 10.6 | 10.9 | 11.2 | 11.5 | 11.8 | 12.1 | 12.4 | 12.7 | 13.0 | 13.3 |

| 5.3 | 5.5 | 5.7 | 5.8 | 6.0 | 6.2 | 6.3 | 6.5 | 6.7 | 6.8 | 7.0 | 7.1 | 7.3 |
|---|---|---|---|---|---|---|---|---|---|---|---|---|
| 10.7 | 11.0 | 11.4 | 11.7 | 12.1 | 12.4 | 12.7 | 13.1 | 13.4 | 13.8 | 14.1 | 14.4 | 14.8 |
| 9.7 | 10.0 | 10.3 | 10.6 | 10.9 | 11.2 | 11.5 | 11.8 | 12.1 | 12.4 | 12.7 | 13.0 | 13.3 |

| 5.3 | 5.5 | 5.7 | 5.8 | 6.0 | 6.2 | 6.3 | 6.5 | 6.7 | 6.8 | 7.0 | 7.1 | 7.3 |
|---|---|---|---|---|---|---|---|---|---|---|---|---|
| 8.9 | 9.2 | 9.4 | 9.7 | 10.0 | 10.3 | 10.6 | 10.8 | 11.1 | 11.4 | 11.7 | 12.0 | 12.2 |

| 5.8 | 6.0 | 6.2 | 6.4 | 6.6 | 6.7 | 6.9 | 7.1 | 7.3 | 7.4 | 7.6 | 7.8 | 8.0 |
|---|---|---|---|---|---|---|---|---|---|---|---|---|
| 4.4 | 4.5 | 4.6 | 4.8 | 4.9 | 5.0 | 5.2 | 5.3 | 5.4 | 5.6 | 5.7 | 5.9 | 6.0 |
| 3.1 | 3.2 | 3.3 | 3.4 | 3.5 | 3.6 | 3.7 | 3.8 | 3.9 | 4.0 | 4.1 | 4.2 | 4.3 |

| 10.5 | 10.9 | 11.2 | 11.5 | 11.9 | 12.2 | 12.5 | 12.9 | 13.2 | 13.5 | 13.8 | 14.2 | 14.5 |
|---|---|---|---|---|---|---|---|---|---|---|---|---|
| 12.3 | 12.7 | 13.1 | 13.5 | 13.9 | 14.3 | 14.7 | 15.0 | 15.4 | 15.8 | 16.2 | 16.6 | 17.0 |
| 7.3 | 7.5 | 7.7 | 7.9 | 8.2 | 8.4 | 8.6 | 8.9 | 9.1 | 9.3 | 9.5 | 9.8 | 10.0 |
| 10.7 | 11.0 | 11.4 | 11.7 | 12.1 | 12.4 | 12.7 | 13.1 | 13.4 | 13.8 | 14.1 | 14.4 | 14.8 |

**Body weight**

| | KG | 45 | 48 | 50 | 52 | 55 | 57 | 59 | 61 | 64 | 66 | 68 | 70 |
|---|---|---|---|---|---|---|---|---|---|---|---|---|---|
| | Pounds | 100 | 105 | 110 | 115 | 120 | 125 | 130 | 135 | 140 | 145 | 150 | 155 |
| Horseback riding | | | | | | | | | | | | | |
| Walk | | 1.9 | 2.0 | 2.1 | 2.2 | 2.3 | 2.4 | 2.5 | 2.6 | 2.7 | 2.8 | 2.9 | 3.0 |
| Sitting to trot | | 2.7 | 2.9 | 3.0 | 3.1 | 3.3 | 3.4 | 3.5 | 3.7 | 3.8 | 3.9 | 4.1 | 4.2 |
| Posting to trot | | 4.2 | 4.4 | 4.6 | 4.8 | 5.1 | 5.3 | 5.5 | 5.7 | 5.9 | 6.1 | 6.4 | 6.6 |
| Gallop | | 5.7 | 6.0 | 6.3 | 6.6 | 6.9 | 7.2 | 7.5 | 7.8 | 8.1 | 8.4 | 8.7 | 9.0 |
| Horseshoes | | 2.5 | 2.6 | 2.8 | 2.9 | 3.0 | 3.1 | 3.3 | 3.4 | 3.5 | 3.7 | 3.8 | 3.9 |
| Jogging (see running) | | | | | | | | | | | | | |
| Judo | | 8.5 | 8.9 | 9.3 | 9.8 | 10.2 | 10.6 | 11.0 | 11.5 | 11.9 | 12.3 | 12.8 | 13.2 |
| Karate | | 8.5 | 8.9 | 9.3 | 9.8 | 10.2 | 10.6 | 11.0 | 11.5 | 11.9 | 12.3 | 12.8 | 13.2 |
| Mountain climbing | | 6.5 | 6.8 | 7.2 | 7.5 | 7.8 | 8.2 | 8.5 | 8.8 | 9.2 | 9.5 | 9.8 | 10.2 |
| Paddle ball | | 5.7 | 6.0 | 6.3 | 6.6 | 6.9 | 7.2 | 7.5 | 7.8 | 8.1 | 8.4 | 8.7 | 9.0 |
| Pool (billiards) | | 1.5 | 1.6 | 1.6 | 1.7 | 1.8 | 1.9 | 1.9 | 2.0 | 2.1 | 2.2 | 2.2 | 2.3 |
| Racketball | | 6.5 | 6.8 | 7.1 | 7.5 | 7.8 | 8.1 | 8.4 | 8.8 | 9.1 | 9.4 | 9.8 | 10.1 |
| Roller skating (9 mph) | | 4.2 | 4.4 | 4.6 | 4.8 | 5.1 | 5.3 | 5.5 | 5.7 | 5.9 | 6.1 | 6.4 | 6.6 |
| Running (steady state) | | | | | | | | | | | | | |
| (mph) | (min/mile) | | | | | | | | | | | | |
| 5.0 | 12:00 | 6.0 | 6.3 | 6.6 | 7.0 | 7.3 | 7.6 | 7.9 | 8.2 | 8.5 | 8.8 | 9.1 | 9.4 |
| 5.5 | 10:55 | 6.7 | 7.0 | 7.3 | 7.7 | 8.0 | 8.4 | 8.7 | 9.0 | 9.4 | 9.7 | 10.0 | 10.4 |
| 6.0 | 10:00 | 7.2 | 7.6 | 8.0 | 8.4 | 8.7 | 9.1 | 9.5 | 9.8 | 10.2 | 10.6 | 10.9 | 11.3 |
| 7.0 | 8:35 | 8.5 | 8.9 | 9.3 | 9.8 | 10.2 | 10.6 | 11.0 | 11.5 | 11.9 | 12.3 | 12.8 | 13.2 |
| 8.0 | 7:30 | 9.7 | 10.2 | 10.7 | 11.2 | 11.6 | 12.1 | 12.6 | 13.1 | 13.6 | 14.1 | 14.6 | 15.1 |
| 9.0 | 6:40 | 10.8 | 11.3 | 11.9 | 12.4 | 12.9 | 13.5 | 14.0 | 14.6 | 15.1 | 15.7 | 16.2 | 16.8 |
| 10.0 | 6:00 | 12.1 | 12.7 | 13.3 | 13.9 | 14.5 | 15.1 | 15.7 | 16.4 | 17.0 | 17.6 | 18.2 | 18.8 |
| 11.0 | 5:28 | 13.3 | 14.0 | 14.6 | 15.3 | 16.0 | 16.7 | 17.3 | 18.0 | 18.7 | 19.4 | 20.0 | 20.7 |
| 12.0 | 5:00 | 14.5 | 15.2 | 16.0 | 16.7 | 17.4 | 18.2 | 18.9 | 19.7 | 20.4 | 21.1 | 21.9 | 22.6 |
| Sailing, small boat | | 2.7 | 2.9 | 3.0 | 3.1 | 3.3 | 3.4 | 3.5 | 3.7 | 3.8 | 3.9 | 4.1 | 4.2 |
| Skating, ice (9 mph) | | 4.2 | 4.4 | 4.6 | 4.8 | 5.1 | 5.2 | 5.5 | 5.7 | 5.9 | 6.1 | 6.4 | 6.6 |
| Skiing, cross country | | | | | | | | | | | | | |
| (mph) | (min/mile) | | | | | | | | | | | | |
| 2.5 | 24:00 | 5.0 | 5.2 | 5.5 | 5.7 | 6.0 | 6.2 | 6.5 | 6.7 | 7.0 | 7.2 | 7.5 | 7.8 |
| 4.0 | 15:00 | 6.5 | 6.8 | 7.2 | 7.5 | 7.8 | 8.2 | 8.5 | 8.8 | 9.2 | 9.5 | 9.9 | 10.2 |
| 5.0 | 12:00 | 7.7 | 8.0 | 8.4 | 8.8 | 9.2 | 9.6 | 10.0 | 10.4 | 10.8 | 11.1 | 11.5 | 11.9 |

| 73 | 75 | 77 | 80 | 82 | 84 | 86 | 89 | 91 | 93 | 95 | 98 | 100 |
|---|---|---|---|---|---|---|---|---|---|---|---|---|
| 160 | 165 | 170 | 175 | 180 | 185 | 190 | 195 | 200 | 205 | 210 | 215 | 220 |
| 3.1 | 3.2 | 3.3 | 3.4 | 3.5 | 3.6 | 3.7 | 3.8 | 3.9 | 4.0 | 4.1 | 4.2 | 4.3 |
| 4.4 | 4.5 | 4.6 | 4.8 | 4.9 | 5.0 | 5.2 | 5.3 | 5.4 | 5.6 | 5.7 | 5.9 | 6.0 |
| 6.8 | 7.0 | 7.2 | 7.4 | 7.6 | 7.9 | 8.1 | 8.3 | 8.5 | 8.7 | 8.9 | 9.1 | 9.4 |
| 9.3 | 9.5 | 9.8 | 10.1 | 10.4 | 10.7 | 11.0 | 11.3 | 11.6 | 11.9 | 12.2 | 12.5 | 12.8 |
| 4.0 | 4.2 | 4.3 | 4.4 | 4.5 | 4.7 | 4.8 | 4.9 | 5.2 | 5.2 | 5.3 | 5.4 | 5.6 |
| 13.6 | 14.1 | 14.5 | 14.9 | 15.4 | 15.8 | 16.2 | 16.6 | 17.1 | 17.5 | 17.9 | 18.4 | 18.8 |
| 13.6 | 14.1 | 14.5 | 14.9 | 15.4 | 15.8 | 16.2 | 16.6 | 17.1 | 17.5 | 17.9 | 18.4 | 18.8 |
| 10.5 | 10.8 | 11.2 | 11.5 | 11.8 | 12.1 | 12.5 | 12.8 | 13.1 | 13.5 | 13.8 | 14.1 | 14.5 |
| 9.3 | 9.5 | 9.8 | 10.1 | 10.4 | 10.7 | 11.0 | 11.2 | 11.6 | 11.9 | 12.2 | 12.5 | 12.8 |
| 2.4 | 2.5 | 2.6 | 2.6 | 2.7 | 2.8 | 2.9 | 2.9 | 3.0 | 3.1 | 3.2 | 3.2 | 3.3 |
| 10.4 | 10.7 | 11.1 | 11.4 | 11.7 | 12.0 | 12.4 | 12.7 | 13.0 | 13.4 | 13.7 | 14.0 | 14.4 |
| 6.8 | 7.0 | 7.2 | 7.4 | 7.6 | 7.9 | 8.1 | 8.3 | 8.5 | 8.7 | 8.9 | 9.1 | 9.4 |
| 9.7 | 10.0 | 10.3 | 10.6 | 10.9 | 11.2 | 11.6 | 11.9 | 12.2 | 12.5 | 12.8 | 13.1 | 13.4 |
| 10.7 | 11.1 | 11.4 | 11.7 | 12.1 | 12.4 | 12.8 | 13.1 | 13.4 | 13.8 | 14.1 | 14.5 | 14.8 |
| 11.7 | 12.0 | 12.4 | 12.8 | 13.1 | 13.5 | 13.8 | 14.3 | 14.6 | 15.0 | 15.4 | 15.7 | 16.1 |
| 13.6 | 14.1 | 14.5 | 14.9 | 15.4 | 15.8 | 16.2 | 16.6 | 17.1 | 17.5 | 17.9 | 18.4 | 18.8 |
| 15.6 | 16.1 | 16.6 | 17.1 | 17.6 | 18.1 | 18.5 | 19.0 | 19.5 | 20.0 | 20.5 | 21.0 | 21.5 |
| 17.3 | 17.9 | 18.4 | 19.0 | 19.5 | 20.1 | 20.6 | 21.2 | 21.7 | 22.2 | 22.8 | 23.3 | 23.9 |
| 19.4 | 20.0 | 20.7 | 21.3 | 21.9 | 22.5 | 23.1 | 23.7 | 24.2 | 24.8 | 25.4 | 26.0 | 26.7 |
| 21.4 | 22.1 | 22.7 | 23.4 | 24.1 | 24.8 | 25.4 | 26.1 | 26.8 | 27.5 | 28.1 | 28.8 | 29.5 |
| 23.3 | 24.1 | 24.8 | 25.6 | 26.3 | 27.0 | 27.8 | 28.5 | 29.2 | 30.0 | 30.7 | 31.5 | 32.2 |
| 4.4 | 4.5 | 4.6 | 4.8 | 4.9 | 5.0 | 5.2 | 5.3 | 5.4 | 5.6 | 5.7 | 5.9 | 6.0 |
| 6.8 | 7.0 | 7.2 | 7.4 | 7.6 | 7.9 | 8.1 | 8.3 | 8.5 | 8.7 | 8.9 | 9.1 | 9.4 |
| 8.0 | 8.3 | 8.5 | 8.8 | 9.0 | 9.3 | 9.5 | 9.8 | 10.0 | 10.3 | 10.6 | 10.8 | 11.1 |
| 10.5 | 10.9 | 11.2 | 11.5 | 11.9 | 12.2 | 12.5 | 12.9 | 13.2 | 13.5 | 13.8 | 14.2 | 14.5 |
| 12.3 | 12.7 | 13.1 | 13.5 | 13.9 | 14.3 | 14.7 | 15.0 | 15.4 | 15.8 | 16.2 | 16.6 | 17.0 |

**Body weight**

| | | | | | | | | | | | | |
|---|---|---|---|---|---|---|---|---|---|---|---|---|
| KG | 45 | 48 | 50 | 52 | 55 | 57 | 59 | 61 | 64 | 66 | 68 | 70 |
| Pounds | 100 | 105 | 110 | 115 | 120 | 125 | 130 | 135 | 140 | 145 | 150 | 155 |
| Skiing, downhill | 6.5 | 6.8 | 7.2 | 7.5 | 7.8 | 8.2 | 8.5 | 8.8 | 9.2 | 9.5 | 9.9 | 10.2 |
| Soccer | 5.9 | 6.2 | 6.6 | 6.9 | 7.2 | 7.5 | 7.8 | 8.1 | 8.4 | 8.7 | 9.0 | 9.3 |
| Squash | | | | | | | | | | | | |
| Normal | 6.7 | 7.0 | 7.3 | 7.7 | 8.0 | 8.4 | 8.7 | 9.1 | 9.5 | 9.8 | 10.1 | 10.5 |
| Competition | 7.7 | 8.0 | 8.4 | 8.8 | 9.2 | 9.6 | 10.0 | 10.4 | 10.8 | 11.1 | 11.5 | 11.9 |
| Swimming (yards/min) | | | | | | | | | | | | |
| Backstroke | | | | | | | | | | | | |
| 25 | 2.5 | 2.6 | 2.8 | 2.9 | 3.0 | 3.1 | 3.3 | 3.4 | 3.5 | 3.7 | 3.8 | 3.9 |
| 30 | 3.5 | 3.7 | 3.9 | 4.1 | 4.2 | 4.4 | 4.6 | 4.8 | 4.9 | 5.1 | 5.3 | 5.5 |
| 35 | 4.5 | 4.7 | 5.0 | 5.2 | 5.4 | 5.6 | 5.9 | 6.1 | 6.3 | 6.6 | 6.8 | 7.0 |
| 40 | 5.5 | 5.8 | 6.1 | 6.4 | 6.6 | 6.9 | 7.2 | 7.5 | 7.8 | 8.0 | 8.3 | 8.6 |
| Breaststroke | | | | | | | | | | | | |
| 20 | 3.1 | 3.3 | 3.5 | 3.6 | 3.8 | 4.0 | 4.1 | 4.3 | 4.5 | 4.6 | 4.8 | 4.9 |
| 30 | 4.7 | 5.0 | 5.2 | 5.4 | 5.7 | 5.9 | 6.2 | 6.4 | 6.7 | 6.9 | 7.1 | 7.4 |
| 40 | 6.3 | 6.7 | 7.0 | 7.3 | 7.6 | 8.0 | 8.3 | 8.6 | 8.9 | 9.3 | 9.6 | 9.9 |
| Front crawl | | | | | | | | | | | | |
| 20 | 3.1 | 3.3 | 3.5 | 3.6 | 3.8 | 4.0 | 4.1 | 4.3 | 4.5 | 4.6 | 4.8 | 4.9 |
| 25 | 4.0 | 4.2 | 4.4 | 4.6 | 4.8 | 5.0 | 5.2 | 5.4 | 5.6 | 5.8 | 6.0 | 6.2 |
| 35 | 4.8 | 5.1 | 5.4 | 5.6 | 5.9 | 6.1 | 6.4 | 6.6 | 6.8 | 7.0 | 7.3 | 7.5 |
| 45 | 5.7 | 6.0 | 6.3 | 6.6 | 6.9 | 7.2 | 7.5 | 7.8 | 8.1 | 8.4 | 8.7 | 9.0 |
| 50 | 7.0 | 7.4 | 7.7 | 8.1 | 8.5 | 8.8 | 9.2 | 9.5 | 9.9 | 10.3 | 10.6 | 11.0 |
| Table tennis | 3.4 | 3.6 | 3.8 | 4.0 | 4.1 | 4.3 | 4.5 | 4.7 | 4.8 | 5.0 | 5.2 | 5.4 |
| Tennis | | | | | | | | | | | | |
| Singles, recreational | 5.0 | 5.2 | 5.5 | 5.7 | 6.0 | 6.2 | 6.5 | 6.7 | 7.0 | 7.2 | 7.5 | 7.8 |
| Doubles, recreational | 3.4 | 3.6 | 3.8 | 4.0 | 4.1 | 4.3 | 4.5 | 4.7 | 4.8 | 5.0 | 5.2 | 5.4 |
| Competition | 6.4 | 6.7 | 7.1 | 7.4 | 7.7 | 8.1 | 8.4 | 8.7 | 9.1 | 9.4 | 9.8 | 10.1 |
| Volleyball | | | | | | | | | | | | |
| Moderate, recreational | 2.9 | 3.0 | 3.2 | 3.3 | 3.5 | 3.6 | 3.8 | 3.9 | 4.1 | 4.2 | 4.4 | 4.5 |
| Vigorous, competition | 6.5 | 6.8 | 7.1 | 7.5 | 7.8 | 8.1 | 8.4 | 8.8 | 9.1 | 9.4 | 9.8 | 10.1 |

| 73 | 75 | 77 | 80 | 82 | 84 | 86 | 89 | 91 | 93 | 95 | 98 | 100 |
|---|---|---|---|---|---|---|---|---|---|---|---|---|
| 160 | 165 | 170 | 175 | 180 | 185 | 190 | 195 | 200 | 205 | 210 | 215 | 220 |
| 10.5 | 10.9 | 11.2 | 11.5 | 11.9 | 12.2 | 12.5 | 12.9 | 13.2 | 13.5 | 13.8 | 14.2 | 14.5 |
| 9.6 | 9.9 | 10.2 | 10.5 | 10.8 | 11.1 | 11.4 | 11.7 | 12.0 | 12.3 | 12.6 | 12.9 | 13.2 |
| | | | | | | | | | | | | |
| 10.8 | 11.2 | 11.5 | 11.8 | 12.2 | 12.5 | 12.9 | 13.2 | 13.5 | 13.9 | 14.2 | 14.6 | 14.9 |
| 12.3 | 12.7 | 13.1 | 13.5 | 13.9 | 14.3 | 14.7 | 15.0 | 15.4 | 15.8 | 16.2 | 16.6 | 17.0 |
| | | | | | | | | | | | | |
| 4.0 | 4.2 | 4.3 | 4.4 | 4.5 | 4.7 | 4.8 | 4.9 | 5.1 | 5.2 | 5.3 | 5.4 | 5.6 |
| 5.6 | 5.8 | 6.0 | 6.2 | 6.4 | 6.5 | 6.7 | 6.9 | 7.1 | 7.2 | 7.4 | 7.6 | 7.8 |
| 7.3 | 7.5 | 7.7 | 7.9 | 8.2 | 8.4 | 8.6 | 8.9 | 9.1 | 9.3 | 9.5 | 9.8 | 10.0 |
| 8.9 | 9.2 | 9.4 | 9.7 | 10.0 | 10.3 | 10.6 | 10.8 | 11.1 | 11.4 | 11.7 | 12.0 | 12.2 |
| | | | | | | | | | | | | |
| 5.1 | 5.3 | 5.4 | 5.6 | 5.7 | 5.9 | 6.0 | 6.2 | 6.4 | 6.5 | 6.7 | 6.9 | 7.0 |
| 7.6 | 7.9 | 8.1 | 8.3 | 8.6 | 8.8 | 9.1 | 9.3 | 9.5 | 9.8 | 10.0 | 10.3 | 10.5 |
| 10.2 | 10.5 | 10.9 | 11.2 | 11.5 | 11.9 | 12.2 | 12.5 | 12.8 | 13.1 | 13.5 | 13.8 | 14.1 |
| | | | | | | | | | | | | |
| 5.1 | 5.3 | 5.4 | 5.6 | 5.7 | 5.9 | 6.0 | 6.2 | 6.4 | 6.5 | 6.7 | 6.9 | 7.0 |
| 6.4 | 6.6 | 6.8 | 7.0 | 7.2 | 7.4 | 7.6 | 7.8 | 8.0 | 8.2 | 8.4 | 8.6 | 8.8 |
| 7.8 | 8.0 | 8.3 | 8.5 | 8.8 | 9.0 | 9.2 | 9.4 | 9.7 | 9.9 | 10.2 | 10.4 | 10.7 |
| 9.3 | 9.5 | 9.8 | 10.1 | 10.4 | 10.7 | 11.0 | 11.3 | 11.6 | 11.9 | 12.2 | 12.5 | 12.8 |
| 11.3 | 11.7 | 12.0 | 12.4 | 12.8 | 13.1 | 13.5 | 13.8 | 14.2 | 14.5 | 14.9 | 15.2 | 15.6 |
| 5.5 | 5.7 | 5.9 | 6.1 | 6.3 | 6.4 | 6.6 | 6.8 | 7.0 | 7.1 | 7.3 | 7.5 | 7.7 |
| | | | | | | | | | | | | |
| 8.0 | 8.3 | 8.5 | 8.8 | 9.0 | 9.3 | 9.5 | 9.8 | 10.0 | 10.3 | 10.6 | 10.8 | 11.1 |
| 5.5 | 5.7 | 5.9 | 6.1 | 6.3 | 6.4 | 6.6 | 6.8 | 7.0 | 7.1 | 7.3 | 7.5 | 7.7 |
| 10.4 | 10.8 | 11.1 | 11.4 | 11.8 | 12.1 | 12.4 | 12.8 | 13.1 | 13.4 | 13.7 | 14.1 | 14.4 |
| | | | | | | | | | | | | |
| 4.7 | 4.8 | 5.0 | 5.1 | 5.3 | 5.4 | 5.6 | 5.7 | 5.9 | 6.0 | 6.1 | 6.3 | 6.4 |
| 10.4 | 10.7 | 11.1 | 11.4 | 11.7 | 12.0 | 12.4 | 12.7 | 13.0 | 13.4 | 13.7 | 14.0 | 14.4 |

**Body weight**

| | | KG | 45 | 48 | 50 | 52 | 55 | 57 | 59 | 61 | 64 | 66 | 68 | 70 |
|---|---|---|---|---|---|---|---|---|---|---|---|---|---|---|
| | | Pounds | 100 | 105 | 110 | 115 | 120 | 125 | 130 | 135 | 140 | 145 | 150 | 155 |

Walking

| (mph) | (min/mile) | | | | | | | | | | | | | |
|---|---|---|---|---|---|---|---|---|---|---|---|---|---|---|
| 1.0 | 60:00 | 1.5 | 1.6 | 1.7 | 1.8 | 1.8 | 1.9 | 2.0 | 2.1 | 2.2 | 2.2 | 2.3 | 2.4 |
| 2.0 | 30:00 | 2.1 | 2.2 | 2.3 | 2.4 | 2.5 | 2.6 | 2.8 | 2.9 | 3.0 | 3.1 | 3.2 | 3.3 |
| 2.3 | 26:00 | 2.3 | 2.4 | 2.5 | 2.7 | 2.8 | 2.9 | 3.0 | 3.1 | 3.2 | 3.4 | 3.5 | 3.6 |
| 3.0 | 20.00 | 2.7 | 2.9 | 3.0 | 3.1 | 3.3 | 3.4 | 3.5 | 3.7 | 3.8 | 3.9 | 4.1 | 4.2 |
| 3.2 | 18:45 | 3.1 | 3.3 | 3.4 | 3.6 | 3.8 | 4.0 | 4.1 | 4.3 | 4.4 | 4.5 | 4.7 | 4.8 |
| 3.5 | 17:10 | 3.3 | 3.5 | 3.7 | 3.9 | 4.0 | 4.2 | 4.4 | 4.6 | 4.7 | 4.9 | 5.1 | 5.3 |
| 4.0 | 15:00 | 4.2 | 4.4 | 4.6 | 4.8 | 5.1 | 5.3 | 5.5 | 5.7 | 5.9 | 6.1 | 6.4 | 6.6 |
| 4.5 | 13:20 | 4.7 | 5.0 | 5.2 | 5.4 | 5.7 | 5.9 | 6.2 | 6.4 | 6.7 | 6.9 | 7.1 | 7.4 |
| 5.0 | 12:00 | 5.4 | 5.7 | 6.0 | 6.3 | 6.5 | 6.8 | 7.1 | 7.4 | 7.7 | 7.9 | 8.2 | 8.4 |
| 5.4 | 11:10 | 6.2 | 6.6 | 6.9 | 7.2 | 7.5 | 7.9 | 8.2 | 8.5 | 8.8 | 9.2 | 9.5 | 9.8 |
| 5.8 | 10:20 | 7.7 | 8.0 | 8.4 | 8.8 | 9.2 | 9.6 | 10.0 | 10.4 | 10.8 | 11.1 | 11.5 | 11.9 |

| | | | | | | | | | | | | | | |
|---|---|---|---|---|---|---|---|---|---|---|---|---|---|
| Water skiing | 5.0 | 5.2 | 5.5 | 5.7 | 6.0 | 6.2 | 6.5 | 6.7 | 7.0 | 7.2 | 7.5 | 7.8 |
| Weight training | 5.2 | 5.4 | 5.7 | 6.0 | 6.2 | 6.5 | 6.8 | 7.0 | 7.3 | 7.6 | 7.8 | 8.1 |
| Wrestling | 8.5 | 8.9 | 9.3 | 9.8 | 10.2 | 10.6 | 11.0 | 11.5 | 11.9 | 12.3 | 12.8 | 13.2 |

| 73 | 75 | 77 | 80 | 82 | 84 | 86 | 89 | 91 | 93 | 95 | 98 | 100 |
|----|----|----|----|----|----|----|----|----|----|----|----|-----|
| 160 | 165 | 170 | 175 | 180 | 185 | 190 | 195 | 200 | 205 | 210 | 215 | 220 |
| 2.4 | 2.5 | 2.6 | 2.7 | 2.8 | 2.9 | 2.9 | 3.0 | 3.1 | 3.2 | 3.2 | 3.3 | 3.4 |
| 3.4 | 3.5 | 3.6 | 3.7 | 3.9 | 4.0 | 4.1 | 4.2 | 4.3 | 4.4 | 4.5 | 4.6 | 4.7 |
| 3.7 | 3.8 | 4.0 | 4.1 | 4.2 | 4.3 | 4.4 | 4.5 | 4.7 | 4.8 | 4.9 | 5.0 | 5.1 |
| 4.4 | 4.5 | 4.6 | 4.8 | 4.9 | 5.0 | 5.2 | 5.3 | 5.4 | 5.6 | 5.7 | 5.9 | 6.0 |
| 5.0 | 5.2 | 5.3 | 5.5 | 5.6 | 5.8 | 5.9 | 6.1 | 6.3 | 6.4 | 6.6 | 6.8 | 6.9 |
| 5.4 | 5.6 | 5.8 | 6.0 | 6.2 | 6.3 | 6.5 | 6.7 | 6.9 | 7.0 | 7.2 | 7.4 | 7.6 |
| 6.8 | 7.0 | 7.2 | 7.4 | 7.6 | 7.9 | 8.1 | 8.3 | 8.5 | 8.7 | 8.9 | 9.1 | 9.4 |
| 7.6 | 7.9 | 8.1 | 8.3 | 8.6 | 8.8 | 9.1 | 9.3 | 9.5 | 9.8 | 10.0 | 10.3 | 10.5 |
| 8.7 | 9.0 | 9.2 | 9.5 | 9.8 | 10.1 | 10.4 | 10.6 | 10.9 | 11.2 | 11.5 | 11.8 | 12.0 |
| 10.1 | 10.4 | 10.8 | 11.1 | 11.4 | 11.8 | 12.1 | 12.4 | 12.7 | 13.0 | 13.4 | 13.7 | 14.0 |
| 12.3 | 12.7 | 13.1 | 13.5 | 13.9 | 14.3 | 14.7 | 15.0 | 15.4 | 15.8 | 16.2 | 16.6 | 17.0 |
| 8.0 | 8.3 | 8.5 | 8.8 | 9.0 | 9.3 | 9.5 | 9.8 | 10.0 | 10.3 | 10.6 | 10.8 | 11.1 |
| 8.3 | 8.6 | 8.9 | 9.1 | 9.4 | 9.7 | 9.9 | 10.2 | 10.5 | 10.7 | 11.0 | 11.2 | 11.5 |
| 13.6 | 14.1 | 14.5 | 14.9 | 15.4 | 15.8 | 16.2 | 16.6 | 17.1 | 17.5 | 17.9 | 18.4 | 18.8 |

www.ingramcontent.com/pod-product-compliance
Lightning Source LLC
Chambersburg PA
CBHW081721270326
41933CB00017B/3248